Table of Conten

- Chapter 1
  Vitamin K2
- Chapter 2 - Vitamin K2 and Bone Health
- Chapter 3 - Vitamin K2 and Heart Health
- Chapter 4 - Vitamin K2 and Other Health Benefits
- Chapter 5 - Combining Vitamin K2 with Other Nutrients
- Chapter 6 - Developing a Vitamin K2 Health Plan

Chapter 1: Understanding Vitamin K2

Vitamin K2 is an essential but often overlooked nutrient that plays a critical role in maintaining our overall health. Unlike its more commonly known counterpart, Vitamin K1, which is primarily involved in blood clotting, Vitamin K2 has unique functions that are vital for bone and cardiovascular health. This vitamin helps ensure that calcium is properly utilized in the body, directing it to where it is needed most—our bones and teeth—while preventing it from accumulating in places where it can cause harm, such as in our arteries.

Vitamin K2 is part of the larger Vitamin K family, but it stands out due to its specific role in regulating calcium. While Vitamin K1 is found predominantly in leafy green vegetables and is important for coagulation, Vitamin K2 is found in animal products and fermented foods, and it is crucial for guiding calcium into bones and teeth, thereby supporting their strength and density. At the same time, Vitamin K2 helps prevent calcium from depositing in soft tissues like the arteries, which can lead to conditions such as atherosclerosis if left unchecked.

The distinction between Vitamin K1 and K2 is not just in their sources and roles but also in their biological availability and activity within the body. Vitamin K2 is more effective than Vitamin K1 in supporting bone and cardiovascular health, making it a key nutrient that many people may be lacking in their diets. Despite its importance, Vitamin K2 is not as widely recognized or understood, which is why it is often under-consumed.

Understanding the importance of Vitamin K2 and ensuring adequate intake is crucial for maintaining a balanced and healthy body, particularly as it relates to managing calcium and preventing the so-called "calcium paradox," where calcium is deficient in bones but excess in arteries. In the pages that follow, we will explore how Vitamin K2 functions within the body, its role in preventing serious health conditions, and how to ensure you are getting enough of this vital nutrient in your daily diet.

Vitamin K2 plays a multifaceted and critical role in the body, particularly in the regulation and utilization of calcium—a mineral that is vital for both bone strength and cardiovascular health. While calcium is essential, its benefits are heavily dependent on where it ends up in the body. Vitamin K2 acts as a guide, ensuring that calcium is deposited in the right places, such as the bones and teeth, and preventing its accumulation in areas where it could cause harm, like the arteries and soft tissues.

One of the primary functions of Vitamin K2 is to activate proteins that regulate calcium. The most well-known of these proteins is osteocalcin, which is produced by osteoblasts, the cells responsible for bone formation. Osteocalcin needs to be activated by Vitamin K2 to bind calcium effectively and incorporate it into the bone matrix. This process not only strengthens bones but also increases their density, making them more resistant to fractures. Without sufficient Vitamin K2, osteocalcin remains inactive, leading to a scenario where calcium, instead of being used for bone-building, may be misdirected.

Another critical protein influenced by Vitamin K2 is matrix Gla-protein (MGP), which is found in the blood vessels and other soft tissues. MGP's primary function is to prevent calcium from being deposited in the walls of arteries, where it could lead to the development of atherosclerosis—a condition characterized by the hardening and narrowing of the arteries due to calcium buildup. When Vitamin K2 activates MGP, it binds calcium and helps shuttle it away from the arteries, reducing the risk of cardiovascular disease.

The importance of Vitamin K2 in these processes highlights its role as a key factor in the prevention of two major health issues: osteoporosis and atherosclerosis. Osteoporosis is a condition where bones become weak and brittle, often due to insufficient calcium being incorporated into the bone matrix. On the other hand, atherosclerosis is a cardiovascular condition where calcium deposits in the arteries, leading to plaque formation and increased risk of heart attack or stroke. Vitamin K2 helps balance these two processes, ensuring that calcium strengthens bones without compromising cardiovascular health.

In addition to its roles in bone and cardiovascular health, Vitamin K2 is also involved in other physiological processes. For example, it supports dental health by promoting the mineralization of teeth, helping to prevent cavities and tooth decay. Furthermore, emerging research suggests that Vitamin K2 may play a role in maintaining healthy skin by influencing the activity of proteins that prevent the calcification of elastin, a protein that gives skin its elasticity. By preventing calcification, Vitamin K2 helps keep the skin supple and reduces the appearance of wrinkles.

Another intriguing area of research is the potential role of Vitamin K2 in cancer prevention. Some studies have indicated that Vitamin K2 might have protective effects against certain types of cancer, including liver and prostate cancers. While the mechanisms are not yet fully understood, it is believed that Vitamin K2 may influence cell growth and apoptosis (programmed cell death), processes that are often disrupted in cancer cells.

The role of Vitamin K2 in the body extends beyond its interaction with calcium and includes broader implications for overall health and longevity. As a fat-soluble vitamin, Vitamin K2 is stored in the body's fat tissues and works in concert with other fat-soluble vitamins such as Vitamins A and D. This synergy is important, as

Vitamin D helps increase calcium absorption in the gut, while Vitamin K2 ensures that the absorbed calcium is correctly utilized.

Despite its critical roles, many people do not get enough Vitamin K2 from their diet, leading to a deficiency that may go unnoticed until significant health issues arise. Ensuring adequate intake of Vitamin K2 is therefore essential for maintaining a balanced and healthy body, particularly as it relates to managing calcium and preventing the complications that can arise from its mismanagement.

In understanding the role of Vitamin K2, it becomes clear that this nutrient is not just a supplement but a necessary component of a healthy diet that supports strong bones, a healthy heart, and overall well-being. By incorporating sources of Vitamin K2 into your diet and considering supplementation when necessary, you can take a proactive approach to safeguarding your health and preventing the conditions that arise from calcium mismanagement.

The "calcium paradox" is a term used to describe a perplexing and dangerous phenomenon: while calcium is crucial for building strong bones, it can also lead to serious health problems when it accumulates in the wrong places, such as the arteries. This paradox arises when calcium, instead of being directed to the bones where it is needed, is deposited in soft tissues like the arteries, contributing to conditions such as osteoporosis and atherosclerosis simultaneously. Understanding the calcium paradox is essential for grasping the vital role that Vitamin K2 plays in maintaining both bone and cardiovascular health.

Osteoporosis is a condition characterized by weakened bones that are more susceptible to fractures. It often occurs when there is not enough calcium in the bones, which can happen if the body is unable to properly incorporate calcium into the bone matrix. On the other hand, atherosclerosis is a condition in which calcium builds up in the walls of the arteries, leading to their hardening and narrowing. This calcification of arteries can significantly increase the risk of heart attacks, strokes, and other cardiovascular diseases.

The paradox lies in the fact that people who are most concerned about their bone health, often supplementing with calcium and Vitamin D, might inadvertently be increasing their risk of cardiovascular disease if they are not also getting enough Vitamin K2. Without adequate Vitamin K2, the calcium that is absorbed through the diet or supplements might not be effectively directed to the bones and teeth. Instead, it can accumulate in soft tissues and blood vessels, leading to harmful calcifications.

Vitamin K2 acts as a crucial regulator in this process. It activates two key proteins: osteocalcin, which binds calcium and integrates it into the bone matrix, and matrix Gla-protein (MGP), which prevents calcium from depositing in the arteries and other soft tissues. When there is a deficiency of Vitamin K2, these proteins remain inactive, and the body's calcium management becomes disrupted. This can lead to bones becoming weaker (due to insufficient calcium) and arteries becoming stiffer (due to excess calcium).

The calcium paradox underscores the importance of a balanced approach to calcium supplementation and bone health. While calcium and Vitamin D are necessary for maintaining bone density and overall health, their benefits can only be fully realized in the presence of sufficient Vitamin K2. This is because Vitamin D increases calcium absorption from the gut, but it is Vitamin K2 that ensures this calcium is properly utilized within the body. Without Vitamin K2, the increased calcium absorption could lead to more calcium being deposited in the arteries rather than in the bones, exacerbating the risk of cardiovascular problems.

The implications of the calcium paradox are significant, especially in aging populations where both osteoporosis and atherosclerosis are common concerns. Many people unknowingly contribute to this paradox by focusing solely on calcium and Vitamin D supplementation without considering the role of Vitamin K2. This lack of awareness can lead to a false sense of security, where individuals believe they are protecting their bones, while in reality, they might be increasing their risk of heart disease.

Addressing the calcium paradox requires a shift in how we approach bone and cardiovascular health. It highlights the need for a holistic understanding of how nutrients work together in the body. Vitamin K2 is the missing piece of the puzzle that ensures calcium benefits the bones without causing harm to the arteries. For those concerned about bone health, especially those at risk for osteoporosis or cardiovascular disease, ensuring adequate intake of Vitamin K2 is crucial.

Incorporating Vitamin K2 into the diet, whether through food sources or supplements, can help prevent the calcium paradox from occurring. Foods rich in Vitamin K2, such as fermented products like natto, cheese, and certain animal products, should be part of a balanced diet, especially for those who take calcium and Vitamin D supplements. Additionally, understanding the importance of Vitamin K2 can lead to better health outcomes, reducing the risk of both osteoporosis and atherosclerosis.

The calcium paradox serves as a powerful reminder of the intricate balance required in nutrient supplementation and health maintenance. By addressing this paradox through the proper intake of Vitamin K2, we can protect both our bones and our cardiovascular system, ensuring that calcium works for us, not against us.

Vitamin K2, while essential for our health, is not as widely available in the diet as some other vitamins. It is naturally found in certain foods, particularly those that are either fermented or derived from animals. Ensuring an adequate intake of Vitamin K2 can be challenging, especially for individuals who do not regularly consume these specific types of foods. Understanding the best sources of Vitamin K2 is crucial for maintaining sufficient levels of this vital nutrient.

One of the richest sources of Vitamin K2 is **natto**, a traditional Japanese food made from fermented soybeans. Natto is particularly high in a subtype of Vitamin K2 known as MK-7, which is highly bioavailable and has a longer half-life in the body compared to other forms. This means that MK-7 stays active in the body for longer periods, making it an efficient source of Vitamin K2. Despite its potent benefits, natto's strong flavor and slimy texture make it an acquired taste, and it is not commonly consumed outside of Japan.

For those who find natto unappealing, **fermented dairy products** such as cheese, particularly hard cheeses like Gouda and Jarlsberg, are excellent sources of Vitamin K2. The fermentation process used to produce these cheeses increases their Vitamin K2 content, making them a valuable addition to a diet aimed at supporting bone and cardiovascular health. The type of Vitamin K2 found in these cheeses is primarily MK-4, another form of Vitamin K2 that, although it has a shorter half-life than MK-7, still plays a crucial role in activating proteins that manage calcium.

Animal products are another significant source of Vitamin K2, especially those derived from animals that are grass-fed or pasture-raised. These animals accumulate Vitamin K2 in their tissues by consuming grass, which contains Vitamin K1 that is then converted into Vitamin K2. Foods such as butter, liver, egg yolks, and certain cuts of meat from grass-fed animals are rich in Vitamin K2. Among these, organ meats like liver are particularly high in MK-4, offering a concentrated source of this important nutrient.

Egg yolks are a convenient and versatile source of Vitamin K2, particularly when the eggs come from chickens that are free-range or pasture-raised. The diet of these chickens, which typically includes grass and insects, enhances the Vitamin K2 content of their eggs. Incorporating egg yolks into your diet can be an easy way to boost your Vitamin K2 intake.

In addition to food sources, the **role of gut bacteria** in synthesizing Vitamin K2 is an important, yet often overlooked, aspect of maintaining adequate levels of this vitamin. Certain strains of bacteria in the gut can convert Vitamin K1 into Vitamin K2. However, this conversion process varies greatly among individuals and is influenced by factors such as diet, gut health, and the presence of beneficial bacteria. A healthy, balanced gut microbiome is essential for maximizing the internal production of Vitamin K2, and consuming fermented foods like sauerkraut, kimchi, and yogurt can support this process.

While it is possible to obtain Vitamin K2 through diet, supplementation is another option, particularly for individuals who may have difficulty consuming enough K2-rich foods or those with specific health concerns that increase their need for this nutrient. Vitamin K2 supplements typically come in the form of MK-4 or MK-7, with MK-7 being the preferred choice for its longer duration of action in the body. These supplements can be an effective way to ensure adequate intake, especially when dietary sources are insufficient.

It's important to note that while Vitamin K1, found abundantly in leafy green vegetables, can be converted into Vitamin K2 by the body, this conversion is relatively inefficient. As such, relying solely on Vitamin K1 intake to meet your Vitamin K2 needs may not be sufficient, particularly for those at higher risk of bone or cardiovascular issues. Therefore, focusing on direct sources of Vitamin K2, whether through diet or supplements, is essential for ensuring that your body has the resources it needs to manage calcium effectively and support overall health.

Incorporating these sources of Vitamin K2 into your diet can be a simple and effective way to protect your bones and cardiovascular system. Whether through traditional foods like natto and cheese or through supplements, ensuring that you get enough Vitamin K2 is a proactive step towards preventing the health issues associated with calcium mismanagement.

Vitamin K2 deficiency, though not as widely recognized as other nutrient deficiencies, can have significant consequences for health, particularly in relation to bone strength and cardiovascular function. Because Vitamin K2 is essential for directing calcium to the bones and away from soft tissues, a deficiency in this vitamin can lead to a range of symptoms and health issues that often go unnoticed until they become more severe.

One of the most common signs of Vitamin K2 deficiency is **bone-related issues**, particularly an increased risk of fractures and osteoporosis. When the body lacks sufficient Vitamin K2, osteocalcin, the protein responsible for binding calcium to the bone matrix, remains inactive. This means that calcium is not effectively incorporated into the bones, leading to lower bone density and, over time, weaker bones. Individuals with a Vitamin K2 deficiency may experience frequent bone fractures, even from minor falls or injuries, and are at a higher risk of developing osteoporosis as they age.

Another key symptom of Vitamin K2 deficiency is related to **cardiovascular health**. Without adequate Vitamin K2, matrix Gla-protein (MGP), which prevents calcium from depositing in the arteries, remains inactive. This can lead to the calcification of arteries—a process that hardens and narrows them, increasing the risk of atherosclerosis, heart attacks, and strokes. People with a deficiency in Vitamin K2 may not exhibit obvious symptoms early on, but as calcification progresses, they may develop high blood pressure, chest pain, or other signs of cardiovascular disease.

Dental issues can also indicate a lack of Vitamin K2. Since this vitamin is crucial for the proper mineralization of teeth, a deficiency may manifest as increased susceptibility to cavities and tooth decay.

Teeth may become weaker and more prone to damage, as the calcium necessary for maintaining strong teeth is not adequately directed where it is needed.

Joint pain and stiffness are less commonly recognized symptoms of Vitamin K2 deficiency but can be related to the accumulation of calcium in soft tissues, including the joints. This calcification can lead to stiffness, reduced mobility, and pain in the affected areas, symptoms often associated with conditions like osteoarthritis. In severe cases, calcification can also occur in other soft tissues, including the kidneys, leading to kidney stones.

Vitamin K2 deficiency may also contribute to **premature aging** and the development of **wrinkles**. Since Vitamin K2 helps prevent the calcification of elastin—a protein that provides elasticity to the skin—a deficiency can lead to reduced skin elasticity, resulting in wrinkles and sagging skin. This aspect of Vitamin K2's role in the body highlights its importance not just for internal health but also for maintaining a youthful appearance.

For individuals with chronic conditions such as diabetes, a deficiency in Vitamin K2 might exacerbate **metabolic issues**. Emerging research suggests that Vitamin K2 plays a role in glucose metabolism and insulin sensitivity. Therefore, a deficiency might contribute to worsening blood sugar control and an increased risk of complications associated with diabetes.

People at higher risk of Vitamin K2 deficiency include those with **limited dietary intake** of K2-rich foods, such as vegetarians or individuals who consume a diet low in animal products and fermented foods. Additionally, those with **gut health issues** that affect nutrient absorption, such as celiac disease or inflammatory bowel disease, may also be more prone to deficiency, as their ability to convert Vitamin K1 to K2 could be impaired.

Recognizing the symptoms of Vitamin K2 deficiency is crucial for early intervention and prevention of more serious health issues. If you experience any of these symptoms or belong to a higher risk group, it may be worth discussing with a healthcare provider the possibility of a Vitamin K2 deficiency. They can recommend dietary changes, supplementation, or further testing to confirm the deficiency and help you restore your levels to support optimal health.

Understanding and addressing Vitamin K2 deficiency is an important step in maintaining strong bones, a healthy heart, and overall well-being. By ensuring adequate intake through diet or supplements, you can help prevent the conditions associated with this often-overlooked nutrient deficiency.

The story of Vitamin K2's discovery and its journey to recognition in the realm of health and nutrition is both fascinating and somewhat obscure. Unlike many other vitamins that were identified and understood relatively quickly after their discovery, Vitamin K2 spent decades in the shadow of its more well-known sibling, Vitamin K1. However, as research advanced, the unique and critical roles of Vitamin K2 in the body became increasingly clear, leading to a renewed interest in this vital nutrient.

The initial discovery of Vitamin K dates back to the 1920s when Danish scientist Henrik Dam was investigating the effects of a cholesterol-free diet on chickens. He observed that the chickens developed hemorrhages and bled excessively, a condition that could not be attributed to a lack of cholesterol. Dam eventually identified a new compound that was necessary for blood clotting, which he named Vitamin K, derived from the German word "Koagulation." For this discovery, Henrik Dam was awarded the Nobel Prize in Physiology or Medicine in 1943, alongside American biochemist Edward Doisy, who determined the chemical structure of Vitamin K.

For many years, Vitamin K was primarily associated with its role in blood clotting, specifically Vitamin K1, which is abundant in leafy green vegetables. However, in the 1930s and 1940s, researchers began to uncover another form of Vitamin K that behaved differently in the body—this was what we now know as Vitamin K2. Unlike Vitamin K1, which is primarily involved in coagulation, Vitamin K2 was found to have unique effects on calcium metabolism, influencing bone and cardiovascular health.

Despite these early findings, Vitamin K2 did not receive the same level of attention as Vitamin K1. For decades, the scientific and medical communities largely focused on Vitamin K1, given its critical role in preventing bleeding disorders. Meanwhile, the importance of Vitamin K2 in directing calcium to the bones and preventing its deposition in soft tissues remained relatively underexplored.

It wasn't until the late 20th century that interest in Vitamin K2 began to grow, thanks in part to the work of researchers who were studying bone health and cardiovascular disease. One significant contributor to this renewed interest was Dr. Weston A. Price, a dentist and researcher who traveled the world in the 1930s studying the diets and health of various indigenous populations. Dr. Price observed that populations consuming traditional diets rich in fat-soluble vitamins had far better dental health and stronger bones than those consuming modern, processed diets. Although Dr. Price did not identify Vitamin K2 by name, he referred to a mysterious "Activator X," which we now believe to be Vitamin K2.

In the following decades, researchers began to connect the dots, realizing that Vitamin K2 was indeed the "Activator X" that Dr. Price had observed, and that it played a crucial role in preventing both osteoporosis and cardiovascular disease. This shift in understanding led to more focused studies on Vitamin K2, revealing its essential functions in activating proteins like osteocalcin and matrix Gla-protein, which manage calcium in the body.

Further research in the 1990s and early 2000s solidified Vitamin K2's reputation as a key player in health, particularly through studies showing that it could help reduce the risk of fractures and arterial calcification. As a result, Vitamin K2 began to gain recognition not just among scientists but also among health professionals and the general public.

Today, Vitamin K2 is recognized as a critical nutrient that supports bone density, cardiovascular health, dental health, and more. Despite this recognition, many people are still unaware of the difference between Vitamin K1 and K2, or the importance of ensuring adequate Vitamin K2 intake. As research continues, the full extent of Vitamin K2's benefits is still being uncovered, with ongoing studies exploring its potential roles in cancer prevention, metabolic health, and longevity.

The history of Vitamin K2 serves as a reminder of how scientific understanding evolves over time and how essential nutrients can sometimes be overlooked before their full importance is understood. Thanks to the efforts of pioneering researchers and the accumulation of decades of evidence, Vitamin K2 is now firmly established as an indispensable component of a healthy diet and a key factor in preventing the "calcium paradox" that can lead to serious health issues.

In summary, the discovery and recognition of Vitamin K2's role in health have been a long journey, but today, we understand its vital functions in maintaining strong bones, preventing cardiovascular disease, and supporting overall well-being. As we move forward, continued research will likely reveal even more about this important nutrient and its potential to improve our health in profound ways.

Chapter 2: Vitamin K2 and Bone Health

Bone health is critically dependent on the proper utilization of calcium, and Vitamin K2 plays a key role in ensuring that calcium is effectively integrated into the bones. The process of bone mineralization, where minerals like calcium and phosphorus are deposited in the bone matrix to make it strong and dense, is highly regulated and requires the activation of specific proteins. Vitamin K2 is essential in this process because it activates osteocalcin, a protein produced by osteoblasts, which are the cells responsible for bone formation.

Osteocalcin is a non-collagenous protein that binds calcium and helps to incorporate it into the bone structure. However, osteocalcin is only effective when it is in its carboxylated form, which is where Vitamin K2 comes into play. Vitamin K2 facilitates the carboxylation of osteocalcin, enabling it to bind calcium ions tightly and ensure that they are deposited in the bone matrix rather than remaining in the bloodstream or being excreted. This process is vital for maintaining bone density and strength, and without sufficient Vitamin K2, bones can become weak and brittle over time.

The role of Vitamin K2 in bone health is particularly important in preventing osteoporosis, a condition characterized by low bone mass and structural deterioration of bone tissue. Osteoporosis increases the risk of fractures, particularly in the hip, spine, and wrist, and is a major health concern, especially among older adults. Vitamin K2 helps to prevent osteoporosis by ensuring that the calcium we consume through our diet or supplements is directed to the bones where it is needed most.

In addition to osteocalcin, Vitamin K2 also activates other proteins involved in bone health, such as matrix Gla-protein (MGP). While MGP is primarily known for its role in preventing calcium from accumulating in the arteries, it also contributes to bone health by regulating calcium deposition in the extracellular matrix of bones. This dual role of MGP highlights the importance of Vitamin K2 not only in directing calcium to the bones but also in maintaining the overall balance of calcium in the body.

One of the key challenges in maintaining bone health is ensuring that calcium is adequately absorbed and utilized. While calcium and Vitamin D are often emphasized in bone health strategies, without Vitamin K2, the benefits of these nutrients may not be fully realized. Vitamin D increases the absorption of calcium from the gut, but it is Vitamin K2 that ensures this calcium is properly integrated into the bones. Without sufficient Vitamin K2, the increased calcium absorption facilitated by Vitamin D can lead to a paradoxical situation where calcium is deposited in soft tissues rather than in bones, increasing the risk of conditions like atherosclerosis alongside weak bones.

This intricate relationship between Vitamin K2, calcium, and bone health underscores the importance of a comprehensive approach to bone health that includes not only adequate calcium and Vitamin D intake but also sufficient levels of Vitamin K2. By ensuring that Vitamin K2 is present in the diet, we can support the natural process of bone mineralization, reduce the risk of osteoporosis, and maintain strong, healthy bones throughout life.

Understanding the role of Vitamin K2 in bone mineralization offers a clear path to preventing bone-related diseases and supporting overall skeletal health. Whether through diet, supplementation, or both, ensuring adequate Vitamin K2 intake is a crucial step in maintaining strong bones and preventing the complications associated with calcium mismanagement.

When it comes to maintaining strong and healthy bones, the nutrients calcium, Vitamin D, and Vitamin K2 form a crucial triad that works together in a highly coordinated manner. Each of these nutrients has a distinct role in bone metabolism, and understanding how they interact is key to optimizing bone health and preventing bone-related diseases such as osteoporosis.

Calcium is perhaps the most well-known mineral associated with bone health. It is the primary building block of bones, providing the structural strength and rigidity that allows our skeletal system to support the body. Throughout life, calcium is continuously deposited in and removed from the bones in a process known as bone remodeling. This dynamic process is essential for repairing micro-damages to the bone structure, adapting to stressors such as physical activity, and maintaining overall bone integrity. However, for calcium to effectively support bone health, it must be properly absorbed, transported, and deposited within the bone matrix, which is where Vitamin D and Vitamin K2 come into play.

Vitamin D plays a critical role in calcium absorption from the digestive tract. When we consume foods rich in calcium or take calcium supplements, Vitamin D enhances the efficiency of calcium absorption by increasing the expression of calcium-binding proteins in the intestinal lining. This process ensures that a sufficient amount of calcium enters the bloodstream, making it available for bone formation and other physiological processes. Without adequate Vitamin D, the body's ability to absorb calcium is significantly reduced, leading to decreased bone mineral density and an increased risk of fractures.

While calcium and Vitamin D are essential for bone health, their benefits are significantly amplified by the presence of Vitamin K2. Vitamin K2 acts as the director, ensuring that the calcium absorbed by the body is deposited in the bones and not in soft tissues like the arteries. As discussed earlier, Vitamin K2 activates osteocalcin, the protein responsible for binding calcium to the bone matrix, thereby promoting bone mineralization. This action helps to fortify the bones, making them stronger and less prone to fractures.

Moreover, Vitamin K2 plays a crucial role in preventing the calcification of soft tissues, particularly the arteries. Without sufficient Vitamin K2, the calcium absorbed by the body through the efforts of Vitamin D can end up in the wrong places, leading to arterial calcification, a major risk factor for cardiovascular disease. This misdirection of calcium is often referred to as the "calcium paradox," where the same mineral that is essential for bone health becomes a threat to cardiovascular health in the absence of Vitamin K2. Thus, while calcium and Vitamin D are indispensable for bone health, Vitamin K2 is the key nutrient that ensures these minerals are used effectively and safely within the body.

Another important aspect of the relationship between these nutrients is their synergistic effects on overall health. While each nutrient individually supports bone health, their combined effects are far greater. For example, studies have shown that individuals who take both Vitamin D and Vitamin K2 experience better outcomes in terms of bone density and cardiovascular health compared to those who take Vitamin D alone. This synergy highlights the importance of a balanced approach to supplementation and diet, where all three nutrients are provided in sufficient amounts to support optimal health.

It's also important to consider the sources of these nutrients. Calcium can be obtained from a variety of dietary sources, including dairy products, leafy greens, and fortified foods. Vitamin D, on the other hand, is synthesized by the skin in response to sunlight exposure, but it can also be found in foods such as fatty fish, egg yolks, and fortified products.

Vitamin K2, as we have discussed, is found in fermented foods like natto, certain cheeses, and animal products from grass-fed animals.

For individuals who may not get enough of these nutrients through diet alone, supplementation can be an effective strategy. However, it's crucial to approach supplementation with an understanding of how these nutrients work together. For instance, taking high doses of calcium without adequate Vitamin K2 can increase the risk of arterial calcification, while taking Vitamin D without enough Vitamin K2 may lead to the same issue. Therefore, balanced supplementation that includes all three nutrients—calcium, Vitamin D, and Vitamin K2—is essential for supporting bone health without compromising cardiovascular health.

In summary, calcium, Vitamin D, and Vitamin K2 form an interdependent trio that is essential for maintaining strong and healthy bones. While calcium provides the structural foundation for bones, Vitamin D ensures its absorption, and Vitamin K2 directs it to where it is needed most. Together, these nutrients work synergistically to support bone density, prevent fractures, and protect against the calcification of soft tissues, making them indispensable components of any bone health strategy.

To truly understand the impact of Vitamin K2 on bone health, it's helpful to look at real-world examples where this vital nutrient has made a significant difference. The following case studies highlight the experiences of individuals who incorporated Vitamin K2 into their health regimens and saw remarkable improvements in their bone health.

Case Study 1: Sarah's Journey to Stronger Bones

Sarah, a 55-year-old woman, had been diagnosed with osteopenia—a precursor to osteoporosis—following a routine bone density scan. Her doctor recommended increasing her calcium intake and starting Vitamin D supplementation to help slow the progression of bone loss. Despite these efforts, Sarah's subsequent bone density scans showed only minimal improvement, and her risk of fractures remained high.

After researching alternative approaches, Sarah came across information about Vitamin K2 and its role in bone mineralization. She learned that without sufficient Vitamin K2, the calcium she was consuming might not be effectively incorporated into her bones. Encouraged by this discovery, Sarah decided to add a Vitamin K2 supplement to her daily routine while continuing her calcium and Vitamin D regimen.

Within a year of starting Vitamin K2, Sarah's bone density scans revealed a significant increase in bone mass. Her doctor was surprised by the results, noting that her bones were now much stronger than before. Sarah reported feeling more confident in her physical activities, no longer fearing the possibility of fractures from minor falls. Her experience underscores the importance of including Vitamin K2 in any bone health strategy, especially for those at risk of osteoporosis.

Case Study 2: David's Recovery from a Fracture

David, a 68-year-old retiree, suffered a hip fracture after slipping on an icy sidewalk. His recovery was slow, and despite following his doctor's advice on calcium and Vitamin D supplementation, his bone healing seemed to lag behind expectations. Concerned about his slow recovery and the possibility of future fractures, David began exploring additional ways to support his bone health.

Through his research, David discovered the benefits of Vitamin K2 for bone healing and overall skeletal health. He learned that Vitamin K2 could help activate the proteins necessary for effective calcium utilization, potentially speeding up his recovery. With the guidance of his healthcare provider, David started taking a daily Vitamin K2 supplement alongside his existing regimen.

Over the next several months, David noticed a marked improvement in his recovery. His follow-up X-rays showed accelerated bone healing, and his physical therapist observed that he was regaining strength and mobility faster than expected. David attributed much of his progress to the addition of Vitamin K2, which seemed to help his body use calcium more effectively for bone repair.

Case Study 3: Emma's Preventive Approach to Osteoporosis

Emma, a 45-year-old mother of three, had a family history of osteoporosis and was concerned about her own bone health as she approached menopause. With her mother and grandmother both having suffered from fractures due to osteoporosis, Emma wanted to take proactive steps to protect her bones. She was already diligent about her calcium and Vitamin D intake, but she wanted to do more to prevent the same fate.

After consulting with a nutritionist, Emma decided to include Vitamin K2 in her daily regimen. She opted for a supplement that combined Vitamin K2 with Vitamin D, ensuring that both nutrients worked synergistically to support her bone health. Additionally, Emma made dietary changes to include more K2-rich foods like cheese and eggs from pasture-raised chickens.

Over the next few years, Emma regularly monitored her bone density through scans. To her relief, her bone density remained stable, with no signs of the bone loss that had affected her mother and grandmother at the same age.

Emma felt reassured that her preventive approach, which included Vitamin K2, was helping to protect her bones and reduce her risk of developing osteoporosis.

These case studies highlight the powerful role that Vitamin K2 can play in supporting bone health, whether through improving bone density, aiding in recovery from fractures, or serving as a preventive measure against osteoporosis. By ensuring that calcium is effectively utilized within the bones, Vitamin K2 helps to strengthen the skeletal system and reduce the risk of fractures and bone-related diseases.

For individuals concerned about their bone health, particularly those with a history of bone density issues or fractures, incorporating Vitamin K2 into their health regimen can make a significant difference. These real-life examples demonstrate how a holistic approach to bone health—one that includes not just calcium and Vitamin D, but also the often-overlooked Vitamin K2—can lead to stronger, healthier bones and a reduced risk of osteoporosis.

Calcium is widely recognized as a crucial nutrient for bone health, and many people turn to calcium supplements to ensure they are meeting their daily requirements. However, supplementing with calcium without adequate levels of Vitamin K2 can pose significant risks, particularly for the cardiovascular system. The key to safe and effective calcium supplementation lies in the balance and proper regulation of calcium within the body—something that Vitamin K2 is uniquely suited to manage.

When calcium is consumed, whether through diet or supplements, it needs to be absorbed into the bloodstream and then directed to the bones, where it can contribute to bone strength and density. This process is facilitated by Vitamin D, which enhances calcium absorption in the intestines. However, simply increasing calcium absorption is not enough to ensure that it benefits bone health. Without sufficient Vitamin K2, the calcium that enters the bloodstream can end up in places where it does more harm than good.

One of the primary risks of taking calcium supplements without adequate Vitamin K2 is the potential for **arterial calcification**. In the absence of Vitamin K2, calcium can deposit in the walls of arteries, leading to the hardening and narrowing of these vital blood vessels. This condition, known as atherosclerosis, is a major risk factor for heart attacks, strokes, and other cardiovascular diseases. The calcification of arteries reduces their elasticity, making it harder for blood to flow smoothly and increasing the workload on the heart.

The mechanism behind this process involves a protein called matrix Gla-protein (MGP), which is found in the arteries and other soft tissues. MGP's role is to bind calcium and prevent it from depositing in soft tissues. However, MGP needs to be activated by Vitamin K2 to perform this function effectively. When there is insufficient Vitamin K2, MGP remains inactive, and calcium can accumulate in the arteries instead of being directed to the bones. This situation highlights the critical role of Vitamin K2 in preventing the "calcium paradox," where the very mineral meant to strengthen bones ends up compromising cardiovascular health.

Another risk associated with calcium supplementation without adequate Vitamin K2 is the potential for **kidney stones**. Calcium can crystallize in the kidneys, leading to the formation of painful stones. While this is less common than arterial calcification, it is still a concern for individuals who consume high amounts of calcium without the balance provided by Vitamin K2. The activation of MGP by Vitamin K2 also helps reduce the risk of calcium-based kidney stones by ensuring that excess calcium is properly managed and excreted.

Bone spurs are another potential consequence of unbalanced calcium supplementation. These are bony projections that develop along the edges of bones, often in joints, and can cause pain and limit mobility. Bone spurs form when calcium is deposited in areas where it is not needed, a process that can be exacerbated by a lack of Vitamin K2. By directing calcium to the bones and away from soft tissues, Vitamin K2 helps prevent the formation of bone spurs.

For individuals who are supplementing with calcium, it is essential to ensure that their intake of Vitamin K2 is sufficient to support the proper utilization of calcium. This can be achieved through a diet that includes Vitamin K2-rich foods, such as fermented products and animal products from grass-fed sources, or through supplementation. The balance between calcium, Vitamin D, and Vitamin K2 is crucial for maintaining bone health without increasing the risk of cardiovascular disease or other complications.

It's also important to consider that not all calcium supplements are created equal. Some forms of calcium, such as calcium carbonate, are more prone to causing issues like kidney stones or arterial calcification, especially when taken in large amounts without adequate Vitamin K2. Choosing a calcium supplement that is well-absorbed and combining it with Vitamin K2 can help mitigate these risks.

In summary, while calcium is essential for bone health, its supplementation must be approached with caution. Without the protective effects of Vitamin K2, calcium can contribute to the very conditions it is meant to prevent, such as osteoporosis and cardiovascular disease. By ensuring that calcium supplementation is balanced with adequate Vitamin K2, individuals can support their bone health effectively while minimizing the risks associated with unregulated calcium in the body.

Maintaining strong and healthy bones requires more than just consuming calcium. It involves a balanced approach that incorporates key nutrients like Vitamin K2, along with lifestyle practices that support bone density and overall skeletal health. Here are some practical tips to help you optimize your bone health and ensure that your body effectively uses the calcium you consume.

1. Include Vitamin K2-Rich Foods in Your Diet

One of the most effective ways to support bone health is by ensuring your diet includes sufficient amounts of Vitamin K2. Foods that are particularly rich in Vitamin K2 include:

- **Fermented Foods:** Natto, a traditional Japanese dish made from fermented soybeans, is the highest known source of Vitamin K2, particularly the MK-7 subtype. If natto is too exotic for your taste, other fermented foods like sauerkraut, kimchi, and certain types of cheese (such as Gouda and Jarlsberg) also provide good amounts of Vitamin K2.
- **Animal Products from Grass-Fed Sources:** Liver, egg yolks, and dairy products from grass-fed animals are excellent sources of the MK-4 subtype of Vitamin K2. These foods are especially beneficial because the animals have converted the Vitamin K1 from their diet into Vitamin K2.

- **Egg Yolks:** Eggs from free-range or pasture-raised chickens have higher levels of Vitamin K2. Incorporating these eggs into your diet can help boost your intake.

2. Pair Calcium with Vitamin K2 and Vitamin D

Calcium, Vitamin K2, and Vitamin D work synergistically to support bone health. While calcium provides the building blocks for bones, Vitamin D enhances calcium absorption, and Vitamin K2 directs calcium to where it's needed most—your bones. To get the most out of your calcium intake:

- **Take Vitamin D and K2 Together:** If you're supplementing with Vitamin D, consider pairing it with Vitamin K2 to ensure that the increased calcium absorption doesn't lead to

unwanted calcification of soft tissues.
- **Balance Your Diet:** Aim to include sources of all three nutrients in your diet. For instance, a meal that includes fatty fish (for Vitamin D), leafy greens (for calcium), and cheese (for Vitamin K2) provides a balanced approach to bone health.

3. Exercise Regularly

Physical activity is one of the most important factors in maintaining bone density. Weight-bearing exercises, such as walking, running, and resistance training, stimulate bone formation and strengthen the bones. Regular exercise also helps improve balance and coordination, reducing the risk of falls and fractures.

- **Incorporate Strength Training:** Lifting weights or using resistance bands can help build and maintain bone density. Focus on exercises that target major muscle groups, as they provide the greatest benefit to your bones.

- **Engage in Weight-Bearing Activities:** Activities that involve standing and movement, such as dancing, hiking, and tennis, help maintain bone density in the legs, hips, and spine.

4. Maintain a Balanced Diet

In addition to specific nutrients like Vitamin K2, calcium, and Vitamin D, a balanced diet rich in fruits, vegetables, whole grains, and lean proteins supports overall bone health. Nutrients like magnesium, potassium, and Vitamin C also play roles in bone metabolism.

- **Magnesium:** This mineral helps convert Vitamin D into its active form, which aids in calcium

absorption. Include magnesium-rich foods like nuts, seeds, and leafy greens in your diet.
- **Potassium:** Potassium helps neutralize acids that can leach calcium from bones. Bananas, sweet potatoes, and beans are good sources of potassium.
- **Vitamin C:** Essential for collagen production, which provides the structural framework for bones. Citrus fruits, strawberries, and bell peppers are excellent sources of Vitamin C.

5. Limit Factors That Can Weaken Bones

Certain lifestyle factors can negatively impact bone health, so it's important to be mindful of these and take steps to mitigate their effects.

- **Reduce Sodium Intake:** High sodium intake can lead to

calcium loss through the urine. Try to limit processed foods and opt for fresh, whole foods whenever possible.

- **Limit Caffeine and Alcohol:** Excessive caffeine and alcohol consumption can interfere with calcium absorption and bone health. Moderation is key—try to limit yourself to one or two cups of coffee per day and moderate alcohol consumption.
- **Avoid Smoking:** Smoking has been shown to decrease bone density and increase the risk of fractures. Quitting smoking can significantly improve bone health and overall well-being.

6. Consider Bone Health Supplements

If you're concerned that your diet may not provide enough of the nutrients needed for bone health, consider supplements that combine calcium, Vitamin D, and Vitamin K2. These supplements are designed to work together to maximize bone health benefits while minimizing the risks associated with unbalanced calcium supplementation.

- **Choose a High-Quality Supplement:** Look for supplements that provide adequate amounts of all three nutrients in a bioavailable form. If possible, consult with a healthcare provider to determine the right dosage and combination for your needs.
- **Monitor Your Bone Health:** Regular bone density tests, especially as you age, can help you and your healthcare provider track your bone health and make any necessary adjustments to your diet or supplementation routine.

By following these practical tips, you can create a comprehensive approach to bone health that not only strengthens your bones but also protects your cardiovascular system and overall well-being. Incorporating Vitamin K2 into your routine is a key step in ensuring that the calcium you consume truly benefits your bones, helping you maintain a strong and healthy skeletal system throughout your life.

The positive impact of Vitamin K2 on bone health is not just theoretical—it has been demonstrated in the real lives of many individuals who have incorporated this vital nutrient into their health regimens. These success stories highlight the transformative effects of Vitamin K2, especially when it comes to preventing osteoporosis, improving bone density, and enhancing overall quality of life.

Story 1: Helen's Renewed Confidence in Her Health

Helen, a 62-year-old retired teacher, had always been proactive about her health. However, after a routine bone density scan revealed that she was at the early stages of osteoporosis, she found herself worried about her future mobility and independence. Helen's doctor recommended the usual regimen of calcium and Vitamin D supplements, but Helen, eager to explore all options, began researching additional ways to support her bones.

Through her research, Helen learned about the crucial role of Vitamin K2 in directing calcium to the bones and preventing it from accumulating in the arteries. She started taking a Vitamin K2 supplement along with her prescribed calcium and Vitamin D. Over the course of a year, Helen noticed significant improvements in her health. Not only did her follow-up bone density scan show a marked improvement, but she also felt stronger and more active than she had in years. Helen credits Vitamin K2 with giving her the confidence to stay active and maintain her independence as she ages.

Story 2: Mark's Journey to Recovery

Mark, a 70-year-old avid gardener, was devastated when he broke his hip in a fall. The injury required surgery and extensive rehabilitation, and Mark was determined to do everything he could to support his recovery. His physical therapist recommended a balanced diet rich in calcium and Vitamin D, but Mark's wife, who had read about Vitamin K2, suggested adding it to his regimen.

Mark began taking a daily Vitamin K2 supplement in addition to his other medications and dietary adjustments. His recovery was remarkable. Not only did his bone heal more quickly than expected, but his doctors were also impressed by the strength of his other bones, which showed no signs of the thinning often seen in older adults. Mark's experience with Vitamin K2 convinced him of its importance, and he continues to take it to maintain his bone health and prevent future injuries.

Story 3: Emily's Preventive Approach

Emily, a 48-year-old accountant, had seen her mother struggle with osteoporosis in her later years, and she was determined to avoid the same fate. A regular exerciser and health-conscious eater, Emily thought she was doing everything right by taking calcium and Vitamin D supplements. However, after learning about Vitamin K2's role in bone health from a nutritionist, she realized there was more she could do.

Emily began incorporating more Vitamin K2-rich foods into her diet, such as fermented cheeses and eggs from pasture-raised chickens. She also started taking a Vitamin K2 supplement to ensure she was getting enough of this important nutrient. Over time, Emily noticed that her nails and teeth, often early indicators of bone health, were stronger and healthier. She also felt more confident about her bone density, knowing that she was taking comprehensive steps to protect her bones against osteoporosis.

Story 4: Robert's Surprise Improvement

Robert, a 65-year-old former athlete, had always been proud of his physical fitness. However, as he aged, he noticed that his joints were becoming stiffer, and he was experiencing more frequent muscle cramps. Concerned about his bone and joint health, Robert visited his doctor, who recommended increasing his calcium intake. Robert also learned about Vitamin K2 and decided to add it to his regimen.

The results were better than he had hoped. Not only did Robert experience less joint stiffness and fewer cramps, but his overall mobility improved as well. His follow-up bone density tests showed that his bones were maintaining their strength, and his doctor was pleased with his progress. Robert now advocates for Vitamin K2 among his friends, particularly those who are active and want to protect their bones and joints as they age.

Story 5: Linda's Comprehensive Health Turnaround

Linda, a 55-year-old businesswoman, was diagnosed with osteopenia and was at high risk for developing osteoporosis. Her doctor prescribed the standard treatment of calcium and Vitamin D, but Linda wanted to explore a more comprehensive approach. After consulting with a naturopath, she added Vitamin K2 to her regimen and made dietary changes to include more K2-rich foods.

Over the next two years, Linda's bone density not only stabilized but actually improved. Her energy levels increased, and she felt more robust overall. Linda attributes her success to the balanced approach she took, ensuring that her body had all the nutrients it needed to support strong bones. Today, Linda continues to follow this regimen, confident that she is doing everything she can to maintain her bone health and overall vitality.

Summary of Chapter 2

These stories illustrate the profound impact that Vitamin K2 can have on bone health, particularly when combined with other key nutrients like calcium and Vitamin D. Whether used as a preventive measure or as part of a recovery plan, Vitamin K2 has helped countless individuals strengthen their bones, prevent fractures, and improve their quality of life. By ensuring that calcium is directed where it's needed—into the bones—Vitamin K2 plays an essential role in maintaining skeletal health and preventing the complications associated with osteoporosis and other bone-related conditions.

These success stories underscore the importance of a comprehensive approach to bone health, one that includes not only adequate calcium and Vitamin D but also the often-overlooked nutrient, Vitamin K2. As more people become aware of the benefits of Vitamin K2, the potential for improved bone health and reduced risk of osteoporosis continues to grow.

Chapter 3: Vitamin K2 and Heart Health

Vitamin K2 plays a crucial role in safeguarding cardiovascular health by ensuring that calcium, an essential mineral for bones, does not accumulate in the arteries where it can cause significant harm. The primary function of Vitamin K2 in heart health is to activate specific proteins that regulate calcium deposition in the body. Without adequate Vitamin K2, calcium that should ideally be used to strengthen bones might instead contribute to the hardening of the arteries—a condition known as arterial calcification.

Arterial calcification occurs when calcium deposits build up in the walls of arteries, leading to their stiffening and narrowing. This process is a key factor in the development of atherosclerosis, a major cause of heart attacks, strokes, and other cardiovascular diseases. Vitamin K2 prevents this by activating matrix Gla-protein (MGP), one of the most potent inhibitors of arterial calcification. MGP works by binding to calcium that enters the bloodstream, preventing it from settling in the arteries. However, MGP needs to be activated by Vitamin K2 to perform this critical function effectively.

Without sufficient Vitamin K2, MGP remains inactive, allowing calcium to accumulate in the arterial walls. Over time, this can lead to the formation of plaques that reduce the flexibility of the arteries, increasing the risk of cardiovascular events. The role of Vitamin K2 in activating MGP is therefore vital not only for bone health but also for maintaining a healthy heart and circulatory system.

In addition to its effects on MGP, Vitamin K2 also plays a role in activating another protein known as osteocalcin. While osteocalcin is primarily associated with bone health, its activation by Vitamin K2 also contributes to cardiovascular health by ensuring that calcium is properly utilized in the bones, rather than being left to potentially cause harm in the blood vessels.

The protective effects of Vitamin K2 on the heart are further highlighted by its ability to reduce the progression of existing arterial calcification. Studies have shown that individuals with higher levels of Vitamin K2 are less likely to experience the progression of calcification in their arteries, even when other risk factors for heart disease are present. This suggests that Vitamin K2 not only helps prevent the onset of arterial calcification but can also mitigate its advancement, making it a valuable nutrient for both preventive and therapeutic cardiovascular health.

Moreover, Vitamin K2's role in reducing arterial calcification has a direct impact on overall cardiovascular function. Arteries that remain flexible and free of calcification can better accommodate the fluctuations in blood flow and pressure that occur with daily activities. This flexibility is crucial for maintaining healthy blood pressure levels and reducing the strain on the heart, thereby lowering the risk of heart disease.

By preventing the buildup of calcium in the arteries and supporting the proper use of calcium throughout the body, Vitamin K2 offers a natural and effective way to protect heart health. This protection is particularly important for individuals who are at risk of cardiovascular diseases due to factors such as age, family history, or lifestyle choices. Ensuring adequate intake of Vitamin K2, whether through diet or supplementation, is a proactive step towards maintaining a healthy heart and reducing the risk of serious cardiovascular events.

In summary, Vitamin K2 is a key nutrient that plays a vital role in cardiovascular health by preventing the harmful buildup of calcium in the arteries. Through the activation of proteins like MGP and osteocalcin, Vitamin K2 ensures that calcium is properly directed to the bones, keeping the arteries clear and flexible. This not only supports bone health but also provides essential protection for the heart, making Vitamin K2 an indispensable component of a heart-healthy lifestyle.

Atherosclerosis is a progressive condition characterized by the buildup of plaque in the inner walls of arteries, leading to their hardening and narrowing. This process impairs blood flow and can lead to serious cardiovascular complications, including heart attacks and strokes. The development of atherosclerosis is complex and multifactorial, involving inflammation, lipid metabolism, and, importantly, the calcification of arterial walls. Vitamin K2 plays a crucial role in preventing this calcification, making it a key factor in managing and preventing atherosclerosis.

The formation of atherosclerotic plaques begins when the inner lining of the arteries, known as the endothelium, becomes damaged. This damage can be caused by a variety of factors, including high blood pressure, high cholesterol, smoking, and diabetes. Once the endothelium is damaged, it becomes more permeable to low-density lipoprotein (LDL) cholesterol, which enters the arterial wall and becomes oxidized. This oxidized LDL triggers an inflammatory response, attracting immune cells like macrophages to the site of damage.

As macrophages engulf the oxidized LDL, they transform into foam cells, which accumulate within the arterial wall and contribute to the formation of fatty streaks—the earliest visible signs of atherosclerosis. Over time, these fatty streaks can develop into more complex plaques composed of lipids, inflammatory cells, and connective tissue. As these plaques grow, they can restrict blood flow through the artery, leading to symptoms such as chest pain (angina) or, in severe cases, heart attacks and strokes.

One of the most dangerous aspects of atherosclerosis is the potential for plaque rupture. When a plaque becomes unstable, its fibrous cap can break open, releasing its contents into the bloodstream. This can trigger the formation of a blood clot, which can suddenly block the artery and cause a heart attack or stroke. The likelihood of plaque rupture is increased by the presence of calcification within the plaque, which makes it more brittle and prone to breaking.

This is where Vitamin K2 plays a critical role. Calcification within the arteries is not merely a byproduct of aging but a pathological process that contributes to the progression of atherosclerosis. Calcium deposits within the arterial walls can make plaques more rigid and increase the risk of rupture. Vitamin K2 helps to prevent this calcification by activating matrix Gla-protein (MGP), which binds calcium and prevents it from being deposited in the arteries.

Without sufficient Vitamin K2, MGP remains inactive, and calcium can accumulate in the arterial walls, contributing to the formation of calcified plaques. These calcified plaques are particularly dangerous because they are less flexible and more likely to rupture than softer, non-calcified plaques. Thus, Vitamin K2 is essential for maintaining the elasticity of arteries and preventing the progression of atherosclerosis.

Research has shown that higher levels of Vitamin K2 are associated with lower levels of arterial calcification and a reduced risk of cardiovascular events. In populations with higher dietary intake of Vitamin K2, rates of heart disease tend to be lower, suggesting a protective effect of this nutrient against atherosclerosis. Conversely, individuals with low levels of Vitamin K2 are more likely to experience calcification of the arteries, leading to a higher risk of developing atherosclerosis and its associated complications.

It's important to understand that atherosclerosis doesn't develop overnight. It is a gradual process that can begin in early adulthood and progress silently over decades. By the time symptoms appear, significant damage may already have occurred. This makes prevention crucial, and ensuring adequate intake of Vitamin K2 is a vital component of any preventive strategy.

In addition to its role in preventing arterial calcification, Vitamin K2 also supports overall cardiovascular health by helping to maintain healthy blood vessels. By keeping the arteries flexible and free from calcium deposits, Vitamin K2 allows blood to flow more easily, reducing the strain on the heart and lowering blood pressure. This not only helps prevent the onset of atherosclerosis but also mitigates the progression of existing disease.

In conclusion, understanding the process of atherosclerosis and the role of Vitamin

K2 in preventing arterial calcification is essential for protecting heart health. By ensuring that calcium is directed to the bones rather than the arteries, Vitamin K2 helps maintain the integrity and flexibility of blood vessels, reducing the risk of plaque formation, rupture, and the serious cardiovascular events that can result. This makes Vitamin K2 an indispensable nutrient for anyone looking to protect their heart and maintain long-term cardiovascular health.

Scientific research over the past few decades has increasingly highlighted the critical role that Vitamin K2 plays in cardiovascular health, particularly in reducing the risk of heart disease. Multiple studies have demonstrated the effectiveness of Vitamin K2 in preventing arterial calcification, a key factor in the development of cardiovascular disease. By examining these studies, we can better understand how Vitamin K2 contributes to heart health and why it is an essential component of a heart-healthy diet.

One of the most significant studies on Vitamin K2 and cardiovascular health is the Rotterdam Study, a large, long-term investigation that explored the dietary habits and health outcomes of thousands of participants over a decade. The study found that individuals with the highest intake of Vitamin K2 had a significantly lower risk of coronary heart disease and arterial calcification compared to those with lower intake. Specifically, those with high Vitamin K2 intake were found to have a 57% reduction in the risk of dying from heart disease, as well as a 52% reduction in severe arterial calcification. These findings strongly suggest that Vitamin K2 plays a protective role in cardiovascular health, particularly in preventing the calcification of arteries that leads to heart attacks and strokes.

Another important study, known as the EPIC-NL cohort study, further supports these findings. Conducted in the Netherlands, this study followed over 16,000 participants and investigated the relationship between dietary Vitamin K2 intake and the risk of cardiovascular events. The results showed that higher dietary intake of Vitamin K2 was associated with a significantly lower risk of coronary heart disease. The study also found that Vitamin K2, but not Vitamin K1, was inversely associated with the risk of developing heart disease, highlighting the specific importance of K2 in cardiovascular protection.

In addition to these large cohort studies, clinical trials have provided further evidence of the benefits of Vitamin K2 for heart health. One such trial, known as the K2 Heart Study, focused on the effects of Vitamin K2 supplementation in postmenopausal women, a group particularly at risk for both osteoporosis and cardiovascular disease. Over the course of three years, participants who took a daily Vitamin K2 supplement showed a significant reduction in arterial stiffness—a key marker of cardiovascular health—compared to those who did not take the supplement. This reduction in arterial stiffness is crucial, as stiffer arteries are more prone to calcification and less able to accommodate changes in blood pressure, increasing the risk of heart disease.

Another randomized controlled trial investigated the effects of Vitamin K2 on individuals with existing coronary artery disease. The study found that those who received Vitamin K2 supplements had a slower progression of arterial calcification compared to those who did not receive the supplement. This finding is particularly important because it suggests that Vitamin K2 not only helps prevent the onset of arterial calcification but can also slow its progression in individuals who already have cardiovascular disease.

Beyond these specific studies, a growing body of research has explored the molecular mechanisms by which Vitamin K2 exerts its protective effects on the cardiovascular system. These studies have shown that Vitamin K2 activates matrix Gla-protein (MGP), which plays a crucial role in preventing calcium from depositing in the arterial walls. By keeping MGP in its active form, Vitamin K2 ensures that calcium is directed to the bones and not the arteries, thereby reducing the risk of calcification and promoting vascular health.

Additionally, Vitamin K2 has been shown to have anti-inflammatory properties, which further contribute to its cardiovascular benefits. Chronic inflammation is a key factor in the development of atherosclerosis and other cardiovascular diseases. By reducing inflammation, Vitamin K2 helps protect the endothelial lining of the arteries, reducing the likelihood of plaque formation and arterial damage.

In summary, the research on Vitamin K2 and cardiovascular disease provides compelling evidence that this nutrient plays a critical role in heart health. From large population studies like the Rotterdam and EPIC-NL cohorts to clinical trials and mechanistic research, the data consistently show that higher intake of Vitamin K2 is associated with a reduced risk of arterial calcification, coronary heart disease, and cardiovascular events. For individuals looking to protect their heart health, ensuring adequate intake of Vitamin K2 through diet or supplementation is a vital strategy.

Calcium is widely recognized for its essential role in building and maintaining strong bones, but its impact on cardiovascular health is often misunderstood. Over the years, several misconceptions about calcium and heart health have emerged, particularly concerning calcium supplementation.

While calcium is crucial for bone health, taking it without adequate Vitamin K2 can lead to unintended and potentially harmful effects on the cardiovascular system. It's important to address these misconceptions to ensure a balanced approach to calcium intake that supports both bone and heart health.

Misconception 1: More Calcium Equals Better Heart Health

One of the most common misconceptions is that more calcium automatically leads to better heart health. While calcium is indeed necessary for many bodily functions, including heart function, excessive calcium intake, particularly through supplements, can be problematic. Without proper regulation, excess calcium in the bloodstream can contribute to the calcification of arteries. This process, known as arterial calcification, is a major risk factor for atherosclerosis, heart attacks, and strokes.

Calcium's role in muscle contraction, including the heart muscle, is well-established. However, its benefits are contingent upon it being appropriately absorbed and directed within the body. When calcium is not adequately managed—meaning it is not properly absorbed by the bones or excreted by the kidneys—it can accumulate in soft tissues, including the arterial walls. This accumulation stiffens the arteries, reduces their elasticity, and compromises blood flow, leading to an increased risk of cardiovascular disease.

Misconception 2: Calcium Alone Is Sufficient for Preventing Bone and Heart Disease

Another common belief is that calcium alone is sufficient for preventing both bone and heart disease. While calcium is a key component of bone health, its effectiveness in preventing osteoporosis and maintaining cardiovascular health is significantly influenced by other nutrients, particularly Vitamin K2 and Vitamin D. These nutrients work together to ensure that calcium is properly absorbed and directed to where it is needed most—namely, the bones.

Vitamin D enhances calcium absorption in the intestines, increasing the amount of calcium available in the bloodstream. However, without Vitamin K2, this calcium may not be efficiently utilized by the bones and can instead be deposited in the arteries. Vitamin K2 activates proteins like osteocalcin and matrix Gla-protein (MGP), which guide calcium to the bones and prevent it from accumulating in the arteries. Therefore, relying on calcium alone, without adequate Vitamin K2 and Vitamin D, can lead to an imbalance that may harm rather than help cardiovascular health.

Misconception 3: All Calcium Supplements Are Created Equal

Not all calcium supplements are the same, and this is a critical point that is often overlooked. The form of calcium and the presence of other co-factors in a supplement can significantly influence its absorption and effectiveness. For example, calcium carbonate is a common and inexpensive form of calcium supplement, but it is less easily absorbed by the body, especially in individuals with low stomach acid. Calcium citrate, on the other hand, is more readily absorbed and can be taken with or without food.

However, regardless of the form, taking calcium supplements without considering the balance with Vitamin K2 can increase the risk of arterial calcification. The misconception that all calcium supplements are equally effective and safe for heart health ignores the need for a holistic approach to supplementation that includes Vitamin K2 to prevent calcium from being deposited in the arteries.

Misconception 4: Dietary Calcium Intake Is Sufficient to Protect the Heart

Another misconception is that simply consuming a calcium-rich diet is enough to protect both bone and heart health. While dietary calcium is generally preferred over supplements due to its association with whole foods that contain other beneficial nutrients, it is still important to consider the balance of Vitamin K2 in the diet. Traditional diets that are naturally high in Vitamin K2—such as those including fermented foods and animal products from grass-fed sources—help ensure that calcium is properly managed within the body.

Modern diets, however, often lack sufficient Vitamin K2, particularly in regions where processed foods are prevalent, and fermented foods are less common. This imbalance can lead to a scenario where dietary calcium, though necessary, is not effectively utilized, increasing the risk of arterial calcification. Therefore, even with a calcium-rich diet, ensuring adequate Vitamin K2 intake is essential for cardiovascular protection.

Misconception 5: Calcium Supplements Are Safe for Everyone

Finally, there is a widespread belief that calcium supplements are safe for everyone, regardless of age, health status, or existing medical conditions. While calcium supplements can be beneficial for certain populations—such as postmenopausal women or individuals with osteoporosis—they may not be appropriate for everyone. For individuals with certain health conditions, such as chronic kidney disease or a history of cardiovascular disease, calcium supplements can pose risks by contributing to calcification in areas where it is harmful.

It is crucial for individuals considering calcium supplementation to consult with their healthcare provider, who can assess their overall nutrient intake, existing health conditions, and the potential need for supplementation with Vitamin K2 to balance the effects of increased calcium intake.

In conclusion, understanding the relationship between calcium, Vitamin K2, and cardiovascular health is essential for dispelling common misconceptions and making informed decisions about calcium intake. Ensuring that calcium is properly managed in the body requires a balanced approach that includes adequate Vitamin K2, whether through diet or supplementation. This holistic perspective helps protect both bone and heart health, preventing the unintended consequences of unbalanced calcium supplementation.

Incorporating Vitamin K2 into your diet is a crucial step in supporting heart health, particularly in preventing the calcification of arteries that can lead to serious cardiovascular diseases. While Vitamin K2 is less common in typical Western diets compared to other vitamins, it is possible to make simple adjustments to ensure you're getting enough of this vital nutrient. Here are some practical tips and dietary recommendations to help you integrate Vitamin K2 into your daily routine for better heart health.

Focus on Fermented Foods

Fermented foods are among the richest natural sources of Vitamin K2, especially in its MK-7 form, which is highly bioavailable and has a longer half-life in the body. Incorporating these foods into your diet is an effective way to boost your Vitamin K2 intake.

- **Natto:** This traditional Japanese dish made from fermented soybeans is the most potent source of MK-7. While natto has a strong flavor and unique texture that may take some getting used to, it offers the highest concentration of Vitamin K2 available in any food. For those who enjoy it, adding natto to meals a few times a week can significantly enhance Vitamin K2 levels.

- **Fermented Cheeses:** Certain cheeses, particularly those made through fermentation, are excellent sources of Vitamin K2. Gouda, Jarlsberg, and Edam are examples of cheeses rich in MK-7. Incorporating these cheeses into salads, sandwiches, or as snacks can be an enjoyable way to increase your intake.
- **Sauerkraut and Kimchi:** These fermented vegetables are not only good for gut health but also provide a modest amount of Vitamin K2. Including these in your meals as side dishes or

condiments can contribute to your overall intake.

Choose Animal Products from Grass-Fed Sources

Animal products from grass-fed or pasture-raised animals tend to have higher levels of Vitamin K2, particularly in its MK-4 form. This form of Vitamin K2 is more readily absorbed and utilized by the body, making it an important addition to a heart-healthy diet.

- **Egg Yolks:** Eggs from free-range or pasture-raised chickens are a valuable source of Vitamin K2. Adding eggs to your breakfast or using them in cooking and baking can help you incorporate more K2 into your diet. The nutrient is concentrated in the yolk, so it's important to eat the whole egg rather than just the whites.

- **Liver and Other Organ Meats:** Organ meats, particularly liver, from grass-fed animals are among the best sources of MK-4. While organ meats are not commonly consumed in modern diets, they can be highly nutritious. Preparing liver in a variety of ways—such as sautéed with onions or incorporated into pâté—can make it more palatable.
- **Butter and Dairy Products:** Butter and dairy from grass-fed cows are also good sources of Vitamin K2. Opt for organic, grass-fed butter and full-fat dairy products to maximize your K2 intake.

Consider Supplements if Necessary

For those who find it difficult to obtain enough Vitamin K2 through diet alone, supplementation can be a practical solution. Supplements are available in both MK-4 and MK-7 forms, and each offers distinct benefits.

- **MK-7 Supplements:** These supplements are derived from natto and provide a longer-lasting form of Vitamin K2. MK-7 is especially beneficial for long-term cardiovascular protection, as it remains active in the body for extended periods.
- **MK-4 Supplements:** MK-4 is the form of Vitamin K2 found in animal products and is often recommended for its quick absorption and effectiveness in supporting bone and heart health. MK-4 supplements typically require more frequent dosing due to their shorter half-life but are still highly effective.

When choosing a supplement, it's important to consider the dosage and the form that best suits your needs. Consulting with a healthcare provider can help determine the appropriate type and amount of Vitamin K2 supplementation based on your individual health status and dietary intake.

Balance Your Diet with Other Heart-Healthy Nutrients

In addition to focusing on Vitamin K2, maintaining a heart-healthy diet involves balancing it with other key nutrients that support cardiovascular function.

- **Omega-3 Fatty Acids:** Found in fatty fish like salmon, mackerel, and sardines, omega-3s help reduce inflammation and lower the risk of heart disease. Pairing these with Vitamin K2-rich foods can provide comprehensive cardiovascular protection.

- **Magnesium:** This mineral plays a critical role in maintaining healthy blood pressure and preventing arterial stiffness. Foods rich in magnesium, such as leafy greens, nuts, and seeds, should be included in a heart-healthy diet alongside Vitamin K2.
- **Antioxidants:** Fruits and vegetables high in antioxidants, such as berries, dark leafy greens, and cruciferous vegetables, help combat oxidative stress, which can damage blood vessels and lead to heart disease.

Incorporate Vitamin K2 Into Everyday Meals

Making Vitamin K2 a regular part of your meals doesn't have to be complicated. Here are a few simple meal ideas:

- **Breakfast:** Start the day with a scrambled egg or omelet made with pasture-raised eggs, paired with a side of fermented vegetables like kimchi or sauerkraut.
- **Lunch:** Enjoy a salad topped with slices of Gouda or Jarlsberg cheese, and add a dressing made from olive oil and a splash of apple cider vinegar.
- **Dinner:** Prepare a dish with grass-fed liver sautéed with onions, or opt for a grilled fatty fish like salmon, accompanied by steamed vegetables.
- **Snacks:** Keep it simple with snacks like slices of fermented cheese, or enjoy a small serving of natto with a sprinkle of soy sauce.

By integrating these foods into your daily routine, you can naturally increase your Vitamin K2 intake, supporting both bone and heart health in the process.

In conclusion, ensuring adequate Vitamin K2 intake through a balanced diet or supplementation is a practical and effective strategy for maintaining cardiovascular health. By focusing on fermented foods, grass-fed animal products, and potentially incorporating supplements, you can protect your arteries from calcification and support a healthy heart for the long term.

Ensuring adequate intake of Vitamin K2 can have profound long-term benefits for cardiovascular health, significantly reducing the risk of heart disease and enhancing overall quality of life. While the immediate effects of Vitamin K2—such as improved arterial flexibility and reduced arterial calcification—are important, the true value of this nutrient becomes even more apparent when considering its impact over the course of years or even decades.

One of the most significant long-term benefits of maintaining sufficient Vitamin K2 levels is the **prevention of atherosclerosis**, a leading cause of heart attacks and strokes. Atherosclerosis is a slow-progressing condition that can begin as early as adolescence, with calcification of the arteries often going unnoticed until it has reached a critical stage. By activating matrix Gla-protein (MGP), Vitamin K2 plays a vital role in inhibiting the calcification process, keeping arteries clear and flexible. Over time, this reduces the likelihood of plaque formation and arterial stiffening, both of which are major contributors to cardiovascular disease.

In addition to preventing the onset of atherosclerosis, long-term Vitamin K2 intake can also **mitigate the progression** of existing cardiovascular conditions. For individuals who already have some degree of arterial calcification, Vitamin K2 can help slow or even halt the progression, thereby reducing the risk of more severe cardiovascular events. Studies have shown that consistent Vitamin K2 supplementation can decrease arterial stiffness and improve overall vascular function, making it a valuable part of a long-term strategy for managing heart health.

Moreover, Vitamin K2 contributes to maintaining **healthy blood pressure**. As arteries become stiffer and less flexible due to calcification, the heart must work harder to pump blood through the body, leading to increased blood pressure. By preventing calcification, Vitamin K2 helps maintain arterial elasticity, allowing blood to flow more easily and reducing the strain on the heart. This not only helps keep blood pressure within a healthy range but also decreases the risk of developing hypertension, which is a significant risk factor for both heart disease and stroke.

Another long-term benefit of Vitamin K2 is its potential to **reduce the risk of heart failure**. Heart failure often results from a combination of factors, including high blood pressure, atherosclerosis, and other forms of cardiovascular strain. By supporting healthy calcium management and preventing the buildup of calcium in the heart's blood vessels, Vitamin K2 helps maintain the heart's pumping efficiency and reduces the likelihood of heart failure over time. For those with a family history of heart disease or who are at high risk due to other factors, maintaining optimal Vitamin K2 levels can be a key preventative measure.

In addition to its direct cardiovascular benefits, Vitamin K2 also supports overall **longevity and quality of life**. Cardiovascular disease is the leading cause of death worldwide, and its prevention is critical for ensuring a longer, healthier life. By protecting the heart and arteries from the damaging effects of calcium mismanagement, Vitamin K2 helps individuals maintain their cardiovascular health well into old age. This not only extends lifespan but also improves the quality of life by reducing the likelihood of debilitating heart conditions that can significantly limit physical activity and independence.

Furthermore, the benefits of Vitamin K2 are not isolated to the cardiovascular system alone. Because Vitamin K2 also plays a crucial role in bone health, maintaining adequate levels of this nutrient supports both a healthy heart and a strong skeletal system. This dual benefit makes Vitamin K2 a unique and powerful nutrient in the fight against both cardiovascular disease and osteoporosis, two conditions that commonly affect aging populations.

In conclusion, the long-term benefits of Vitamin K2 for cardiovascular health are both profound and far-reaching. By preventing arterial calcification, supporting healthy blood pressure, and reducing the risk of heart failure and other cardiovascular diseases, Vitamin K2 is essential for anyone looking to protect their heart over the long term. Whether through diet or supplementation, ensuring adequate intake of Vitamin K2 is a proactive and effective strategy for maintaining cardiovascular health and enhancing overall longevity.

Chapter 4: Vitamin K2 and Other Health Benefits

Vitamin K2 plays a significant yet often overlooked role in maintaining dental health. While calcium and Vitamin D are commonly associated with strong teeth, Vitamin K2 is essential in ensuring that these minerals are properly utilized to maintain healthy teeth and prevent cavities. By activating proteins that regulate the deposition of calcium, Vitamin K2 contributes to the formation and maintenance of strong, resilient teeth.

Teeth, like bones, require a constant supply of calcium to stay strong and resistant to decay. The process of remineralization, where minerals such as calcium and phosphate are deposited back into the tooth enamel, is vital for repairing early signs of decay and maintaining the integrity of the teeth. Osteocalcin, a protein activated by Vitamin K2, plays a crucial role in this process. When activated, osteocalcin binds calcium and promotes its deposition in the tooth enamel, helping to strengthen the teeth and protect them against cavities.

Without adequate Vitamin K2, osteocalcin remains inactive, and the calcium absorbed through diet or supplements may not be effectively utilized for dental health. This can lead to weaker enamel, making teeth more susceptible to decay and cavities. Additionally, a lack of Vitamin K2 may contribute to the formation of dental plaque, which can further erode the enamel and lead to tooth decay.

Vitamin K2 also helps prevent the calcification of soft tissues, including the pulp and gums, which are critical components of dental health. Calcification in these areas can lead to hardening and reduced function, contributing to periodontal disease and other dental issues. By preventing unwanted calcification, Vitamin K2 helps maintain the health and flexibility of these tissues, supporting overall dental health.

Moreover, Vitamin K2's role in dental health extends to its impact on jawbone density. Just as it supports bone density throughout the body, Vitamin K2 helps maintain the density and strength of the jawbone, which is essential for keeping teeth securely anchored. A strong jawbone reduces the risk of tooth loss and supports the alignment and spacing of teeth, further contributing to overall dental health.

In traditional diets, where fermented foods and organ meats were more commonly consumed, the incidence of dental cavities was significantly lower compared to modern diets. This has been attributed in part to higher levels of Vitamin K2 in these diets, which supported better overall dental health. Today, with the prevalence of processed foods and a decline in the consumption of K2-rich foods, dental health issues such as cavities and gum disease have become more common. Ensuring adequate intake of Vitamin K2 through diet or supplementation can help counteract these trends and support healthier teeth and gums.

For those concerned about their dental health, particularly in the context of preventing cavities and maintaining strong teeth, incorporating Vitamin K2 into the diet is a key strategy. Foods rich in Vitamin K2, such as fermented cheeses, natto, and organ meats, can provide the necessary nutrients to support strong enamel and healthy gums. Additionally, Vitamin K2 supplements are available for those who may not consume enough of these foods in their regular diet.

In summary, Vitamin K2 is an essential nutrient for dental health, playing a critical role in the remineralization of teeth, the prevention of cavities, and the maintenance of healthy gums and jawbone density. By ensuring adequate Vitamin K2 intake, you can support the strength and resilience of your teeth, helping to maintain a healthy, cavity-free smile.

Vitamin K2 is increasingly recognized for its benefits beyond bone and cardiovascular health, with emerging research highlighting its role in maintaining skin health and slowing the aging process. While much of the focus on skincare revolves around topical treatments, the nutrients we consume play a crucial role in the skin's overall health and appearance. Vitamin K2, in particular, contributes to skin elasticity, reduces the appearance of wrinkles, and helps maintain a youthful complexion by influencing the body's use of calcium.

One of the key factors in the aging of skin is the calcification of elastin, a protein that provides elasticity and firmness to the skin. Elastin allows the skin to return to its original shape after stretching or contracting, and it is essential for maintaining a smooth, youthful appearance. As we age, calcium can deposit in the elastin fibers of the skin, causing them to become stiff and less elastic. This process leads to the formation of wrinkles, sagging, and other signs of aging.

Vitamin K2 helps prevent the calcification of elastin by activating matrix Gla-protein (MGP), which inhibits calcium deposits in soft tissues, including the skin. By keeping elastin fibers flexible and resilient, Vitamin K2 helps maintain the skin's youthful elasticity, reducing the appearance of fine lines and wrinkles. This action not only slows the visible signs of aging but also supports overall skin health by preserving the structural integrity of the skin.

In addition to its role in preventing calcification, Vitamin K2 also supports healthy blood circulation, which is essential for maintaining vibrant, youthful skin. Good circulation ensures that skin cells receive the oxygen and nutrients they need to function optimally and that waste products are efficiently removed. By contributing to cardiovascular health and preventing the hardening of arteries,

Vitamin K2 helps maintain healthy blood flow to the skin, promoting a radiant complexion.

Another important aspect of Vitamin K2's impact on aging is its potential role in reducing the appearance of dark circles and bruising. Dark circles under the eyes are often caused by fragile blood vessels and poor circulation, which lead to the pooling of blood and a bluish or purplish tint to the skin. Similarly, bruising occurs when blood vessels break and blood leaks into the surrounding tissues. Vitamin K2 strengthens blood vessels and capillaries, reducing their fragility and helping to prevent the formation of dark circles and bruises. While topical Vitamin K creams are often recommended for these issues, supporting the skin from within by ensuring adequate intake of Vitamin K2 can provide more lasting results.

Vitamin K2 also plays a role in supporting collagen, another critical protein for maintaining youthful skin. Collagen provides the skin with structure and firmness, but its production naturally declines with age, leading to sagging and wrinkles. While collagen is primarily associated with Vitamin C and other nutrients, Vitamin K2 contributes to the overall matrix in which collagen functions, supporting the skin's structural integrity.

Emerging research suggests that Vitamin K2 may also have protective effects against skin cancer. Some studies have indicated that Vitamin K2 can help regulate cell growth and apoptosis (programmed cell death), processes that are often disrupted in cancerous cells. While more research is needed in this area, these findings suggest that Vitamin K2's benefits for skin health may extend to protecting against certain types of skin cancer, further emphasizing its role in maintaining healthy skin as we age.

Maintaining adequate levels of Vitamin K2 can be a powerful tool in a comprehensive anti-aging strategy. By preventing the calcification of elastin, supporting healthy circulation, and potentially protecting against skin cancer, Vitamin K2 helps preserve the skin's youthful appearance and functionality. Incorporating Vitamin K2-rich foods into your diet, such as fermented cheeses, egg yolks from pasture-raised chickens, and natto, can provide these benefits naturally. For those who may struggle to get enough Vitamin K2 through diet alone, supplementation offers a convenient alternative.

In summary, Vitamin K2's impact on skin health and aging is multifaceted, offering protection against the calcification of elastin, supporting collagen, improving circulation, and potentially reducing the risk of skin cancer. These benefits make Vitamin K2 an essential nutrient not just for maintaining a youthful appearance but also for supporting the skin's overall health and resilience as we age.

Vitamin K2 is emerging as a crucial nutrient in the regulation of metabolic health, with significant implications for managing conditions like diabetes and metabolic syndrome. While traditionally associated with bone and cardiovascular health, Vitamin K2's role in metabolism is gaining recognition, particularly for its potential to improve insulin sensitivity and glucose metabolism.

Metabolic health is intricately linked to how the body processes and utilizes nutrients, with insulin playing a central role. Insulin is a hormone that regulates blood sugar levels by facilitating the uptake of glucose into cells, where it can be used for energy. However, in conditions like insulin resistance, the body's cells become less responsive to insulin, leading to higher blood sugar levels and, eventually, the development of type 2 diabetes.

Research suggests that Vitamin K2 may help improve insulin sensitivity, making the body more responsive to insulin and better able to manage blood sugar levels. One way Vitamin K2 supports metabolic health is through its role in activating proteins involved in glucose metabolism. For instance, Vitamin K2 has been shown to influence the expression of osteocalcin, a hormone produced by bones that plays a role in regulating insulin sensitivity and energy metabolism. When activated by Vitamin K2, osteocalcin helps improve the efficiency of insulin, enhancing glucose uptake by cells and reducing blood sugar levels.

In addition to its effects on insulin sensitivity, Vitamin K2 may also help reduce the risk of developing type 2 diabetes by preventing the calcification of pancreatic beta cells. These cells are responsible for producing insulin, and their proper function is critical for maintaining metabolic health. Calcification of the beta cells can impair their ability to produce insulin, leading to higher blood sugar levels and increased risk of diabetes. By preventing this calcification, Vitamin K2 helps protect the pancreas and supports the body's natural ability to regulate blood sugar.

Vitamin K2's role in metabolic health extends to its impact on fat metabolism and weight management. Some studies suggest that Vitamin K2 may help reduce the accumulation of visceral fat, the type of fat that surrounds internal organs and is associated with higher risks of metabolic disorders. This effect is thought to be related to Vitamin K2's influence on adiponectin, a hormone involved in regulating glucose levels and fatty acid breakdown. Higher levels of adiponectin are associated with improved insulin sensitivity and a lower risk of obesity-related complications.

Moreover, Vitamin K2 may play a protective role against the development of fatty liver disease, a condition often linked to obesity and insulin resistance. Fatty liver disease occurs when excess fat builds up in the liver, leading to inflammation and scarring. This condition can progress to more severe liver damage if not managed properly. Vitamin K2 has been shown to help reduce liver fat accumulation, potentially by improving insulin sensitivity and supporting healthy fat metabolism.

Another important aspect of Vitamin K2's impact on metabolic health is its potential role in reducing inflammation, a key driver of many metabolic disorders. Chronic low-grade inflammation is associated with insulin resistance, obesity, and type 2 diabetes. By activating proteins that regulate calcium and reduce oxidative stress, Vitamin K2 helps mitigate inflammation, supporting overall metabolic function.

For individuals managing metabolic conditions like diabetes, ensuring adequate intake of Vitamin K2 can be an important part of a comprehensive approach to health. Foods rich in Vitamin K2, such as fermented products and animal products from grass-fed sources, can naturally enhance K2 levels and support metabolic health. In some cases, supplementation may be necessary to achieve optimal Vitamin K2 levels, particularly for those with dietary restrictions or who are at higher risk for metabolic disorders.

Incorporating Vitamin K2 into a balanced diet, alongside other nutrients that support metabolic health, such as omega-3 fatty acids and magnesium, can help improve insulin sensitivity, regulate blood sugar levels, and reduce the risk of complications associated with metabolic syndrome and type 2 diabetes.

Vitamin K2 is gaining attention for its potential role in cancer prevention, with emerging research suggesting that this nutrient may help reduce the risk of certain types of cancer. While the mechanisms behind Vitamin K2's protective effects are still being studied, there is growing evidence that it plays a significant role in regulating cell growth, promoting healthy cell function, and inducing apoptosis (programmed cell death) in cancerous cells. These actions are critical in preventing the uncontrolled cell proliferation that characterizes cancer.

One of the key ways Vitamin K2 may contribute to cancer prevention is through its ability to regulate calcium in the body. Calcium is not only essential for bone health but also plays a role in cell signaling and the regulation of cell life cycles. Abnormal calcium signaling can lead to uncontrolled cell growth, a hallmark of cancer. By ensuring that calcium is properly managed within the body, Vitamin K2 helps maintain normal cell function and prevents the conditions that can lead to cancer development.

Research has shown that Vitamin K2 can influence the expression of genes involved in cell growth and apoptosis. For instance, studies have demonstrated that Vitamin K2 can activate certain proteins that promote the self-destruction of cancerous cells, effectively preventing them from multiplying and spreading. This process is particularly important in the early stages of cancer, where the body's natural defense mechanisms can often eliminate abnormal cells before they develop into full-blown cancer.

Vitamin K2's role in cancer prevention is supported by epidemiological studies that have found a correlation between higher dietary intake of Vitamin K2 and a reduced risk of certain cancers, particularly liver and prostate cancers. In one study, men with higher intake of Vitamin K2 were found to have a significantly lower risk of developing prostate cancer compared to those with lower intake. This protective effect was especially pronounced in advanced stages of the disease, suggesting that Vitamin K2 may be particularly effective in slowing the progression of prostate cancer.

Similarly, research on liver cancer has shown that Vitamin K2 supplementation can reduce the recurrence of liver cancer in patients who have undergone treatment for the disease. This is thought to be due to Vitamin K2's ability to inhibit the growth of cancer cells and promote apoptosis, helping to prevent the return of cancer after initial treatment. These findings are particularly important given the high rates of liver cancer recurrence and the limited treatment options available.

Another area of interest is Vitamin K2's potential role in preventing lung cancer. Preliminary studies have suggested that Vitamin K2 may help protect against lung cancer by modulating cell cycle regulation and promoting apoptosis in lung tissue. While more research is needed to confirm these findings, the initial results are promising and suggest that Vitamin K2 could play a role in reducing the risk of this deadly disease.

In addition to its direct effects on cancer cells, Vitamin K2 may also contribute to cancer prevention by supporting the body's overall immune function. A strong immune system is crucial for identifying and destroying cancer cells before they can establish themselves and spread. By maintaining cardiovascular health, reducing inflammation, and supporting the proper function of various cellular processes, Vitamin K2 helps create an environment in the body that is less conducive to cancer development.

It is important to note that while Vitamin K2 shows promise in cancer prevention, it is not a standalone cure or treatment for cancer. Instead, it should be considered as part of a broader strategy that includes a healthy diet, regular exercise, and other lifestyle factors that contribute to overall health and well-being. For individuals at higher risk of cancer, such as those with a family history of the disease or those with other risk factors, ensuring adequate intake of Vitamin K2 may offer an additional layer of protection.

Incorporating Vitamin K2-rich foods into your diet, such as fermented cheeses, natto, and organ meats, can help boost your intake of this important nutrient. For those who may have difficulty obtaining enough Vitamin K2 through diet alone, supplementation offers a convenient alternative, especially for individuals looking to enhance their cancer prevention strategies.

In conclusion, while research is still ongoing, the evidence supporting Vitamin K2's role in cancer prevention is growing. By regulating calcium, promoting healthy cell function, and inducing apoptosis in cancerous cells, Vitamin K2 may help reduce the risk of developing certain cancers, particularly liver, prostate, and possibly lung cancer. As part of a comprehensive approach to health, Vitamin K2 offers a promising tool for supporting the body's natural defenses against cancer.

Vitamin K2 is often discussed in the context of bone and cardiovascular health, but its benefits extend to reproductive health as well. Both men and women can potentially benefit from adequate levels of Vitamin K2, which plays a role in hormone regulation, fertility, and overall reproductive function. Emerging research suggests that Vitamin K2 may be an important nutrient for maintaining healthy reproductive systems and preventing conditions that can affect fertility and sexual health.

For women, one of the key ways Vitamin K2 supports reproductive health is through its impact on hormone balance. Hormonal imbalances can lead to a variety of reproductive issues, including irregular menstrual cycles, polycystic ovary syndrome (PCOS), and difficulties with conception. Vitamin K2 helps regulate the production and activity of sex hormones such as estrogen and progesterone, which are critical for normal menstrual cycles and fertility.

In particular, Vitamin K2's role in activating proteins involved in calcium regulation can influence the function of the ovaries, which require a delicate balance of hormones to produce healthy eggs and support conception. By ensuring that calcium is properly utilized and preventing its excessive buildup in the ovaries, Vitamin K2 may help reduce the risk of conditions like ovarian cysts and support overall reproductive health.

Moreover, Vitamin K2's anti-inflammatory properties can be beneficial for women experiencing conditions such as endometriosis, a painful disorder where tissue similar to the lining of the uterus grows outside the uterus. Inflammation is a significant contributor to the pain and complications associated with endometriosis, and by reducing inflammation, Vitamin K2 may help alleviate some of the symptoms and improve quality of life for women with this condition.

For men, Vitamin K2 plays a role in supporting testosterone production and overall male fertility. Testosterone is the primary male sex hormone, and it is essential for the development and maintenance of male reproductive tissues, as well as for the production of sperm. Research has shown that Vitamin K2 can help increase testosterone levels by activating specific proteins in the testes that are involved in hormone synthesis.

Additionally, Vitamin K2's ability to regulate calcium and prevent calcification has implications for prostate health. The prostate gland is prone to calcification as men age, which can lead to benign prostatic hyperplasia (BPH) and other prostate issues. By preventing the buildup of calcium in the prostate, Vitamin K2 may help reduce the risk of these conditions, supporting healthy urinary and sexual function.

Another important aspect of Vitamin K2's impact on reproductive health is its potential role in reducing the risk of reproductive cancers. As mentioned earlier, Vitamin K2 has been shown to influence cell growth and apoptosis, helping to prevent the development and progression of cancer. For women, this may include a reduced risk of breast and ovarian cancers, while for men, it may help protect against prostate cancer.

In addition to these direct effects on reproductive health, Vitamin K2 also supports overall metabolic health, which is closely linked to fertility and reproductive function. Conditions such as obesity, insulin resistance, and metabolic syndrome can negatively impact reproductive health, leading to issues such as reduced fertility, irregular menstrual cycles, and erectile dysfunction. By improving insulin sensitivity and supporting healthy metabolism, Vitamin K2 contributes to a healthier environment for reproductive organs and processes.

For couples trying to conceive, ensuring adequate intake of Vitamin K2 can be an important part of a preconception health plan. Foods rich in Vitamin K2, such as fermented cheeses, egg yolks from pasture-raised chickens, and organ meats, can help provide the necessary nutrients to support reproductive health. In cases where dietary intake may be insufficient, particularly for individuals with dietary restrictions or specific health concerns, Vitamin K2 supplementation may be recommended.

Overall, Vitamin K2 offers a range of benefits for reproductive health, from hormone regulation and fertility support to the prevention of reproductive cancers and conditions like BPH and endometriosis. By incorporating Vitamin K2 into a balanced diet or supplement regimen, both men and women can enhance their reproductive health and increase their chances of successful conception and healthy pregnancies.

Vitamin K2 is a powerhouse nutrient that plays a critical role in various aspects of health, extending far beyond its well-known benefits for bone and cardiovascular health. Throughout this chapter, we've explored how Vitamin K2 contributes to dental health, skin health, metabolic function, cancer prevention, and reproductive health. This final page will summarize these broad-spectrum benefits, reinforcing why Vitamin K2 is an essential component of a healthy diet and lifestyle.

One of the most significant advantages of Vitamin K2 is its ability to ensure that calcium, an essential mineral, is correctly utilized in the body. By activating proteins that regulate calcium, such as osteocalcin and matrix Gla-protein (MGP), Vitamin K2 directs calcium to where it's needed—into the bones and teeth—while preventing it from depositing in soft tissues like arteries and the skin. This precise management of calcium is crucial not only for maintaining strong bones and preventing osteoporosis but also for protecting against arterial calcification, a major risk factor for cardiovascular diseases.

In the realm of dental health, Vitamin K2 supports the remineralization of teeth, helping to prevent cavities and maintain strong enamel. It also plays a role in maintaining healthy gums and preventing the calcification of soft tissues in the mouth, which can lead to periodontal disease. By supporting the health of the jawbone, Vitamin K2 helps keep teeth securely anchored, reducing the risk of tooth loss.

When it comes to skin health and aging, Vitamin K2 is instrumental in preventing the calcification of elastin, a protein that gives skin its elasticity and firmness. By keeping elastin fibers flexible, Vitamin K2 helps maintain a youthful complexion, reducing the appearance of wrinkles and sagging. Additionally, Vitamin K2 supports healthy blood circulation, which is essential for delivering nutrients to the skin and maintaining its vitality.

Vitamin K2's role in metabolic health is another key benefit, particularly its ability to improve insulin sensitivity and support glucose metabolism. This makes it an important nutrient for managing conditions like diabetes and metabolic syndrome. By preventing the calcification of pancreatic beta cells, Vitamin K2 helps maintain their function, supporting healthy insulin production and blood sugar regulation. Its potential to reduce visceral fat and protect against fatty liver disease further underscores its importance in metabolic health.

In the context of cancer prevention, Vitamin K2's ability to regulate cell growth and promote apoptosis in cancerous cells is a powerful defense mechanism. While more research is needed, the existing evidence suggests that Vitamin K2 may reduce the risk of certain cancers, including liver, prostate, and possibly lung cancer. This adds an important dimension to Vitamin K2's role in overall health and disease prevention.

Reproductive health is yet another area where Vitamin K2 shines. For women, it supports hormone balance and may help prevent conditions like polycystic ovary syndrome (PCOS) and endometriosis. For men, Vitamin K2 supports testosterone production and prostate health, potentially reducing the risk of benign prostatic hyperplasia (BPH) and prostate cancer. These benefits make

Vitamin K2 a valuable nutrient for maintaining reproductive health and fertility in both men and women.

In summary, Vitamin K2 is a multifaceted nutrient that offers a wide range of health benefits. By supporting bone and dental health, enhancing skin vitality, improving metabolic function, aiding in cancer prevention, and promoting reproductive health, Vitamin K2 proves to be an indispensable component of a comprehensive health strategy. Ensuring adequate intake of Vitamin K2 through diet or supplementation can help protect against a variety of health conditions and improve overall well-being, making it a key factor in achieving and maintaining a healthy, balanced life.

Chapter 5: Combining Vitamin K2 with Other Nutrients

Vitamin K2 and Vitamin D are two essential nutrients that work together in a synergistic manner to optimize various aspects of health, particularly bone and cardiovascular health. While each nutrient plays a distinct role in the body, their combined effects are significantly more powerful than when they are taken separately. Understanding how these vitamins interact can help you make informed decisions about your health and supplementation routine.

Vitamin D is well-known for its role in promoting calcium absorption in the intestines. It increases the efficiency with which calcium is absorbed from the food we eat, ensuring that there is enough calcium available in the bloodstream for various bodily functions, including bone formation. Without adequate Vitamin D, calcium absorption is significantly reduced, which can lead to weakened bones and an increased risk of fractures.

However, simply increasing calcium absorption is not enough to guarantee strong and healthy bones. This is where Vitamin K2 comes into play. Once calcium is absorbed into the bloodstream, it needs to be directed to the right places in the body, such as the bones and teeth, rather than being deposited in soft tissues like the arteries. Vitamin K2 is crucial for this process because it activates proteins like osteocalcin and matrix Gla-protein (MGP), which help bind calcium to the bone matrix and prevent its accumulation in the arteries.

The synergy between Vitamin K2 and Vitamin D is most evident in their combined effect on bone health. Vitamin D ensures that there is sufficient calcium available in the bloodstream, while Vitamin K2 makes sure that this calcium is effectively utilized for bone formation and maintenance. Together, these vitamins help maintain bone density, reduce the risk of fractures, and prevent osteoporosis.

Moreover, this synergy extends to cardiovascular health as well. By preventing calcium from being deposited in the arteries, Vitamin K2 reduces the risk of arterial calcification—a condition that can lead to atherosclerosis, heart attacks, and strokes. Vitamin D's role in increasing calcium absorption is balanced by Vitamin K2's ability to direct that calcium to the right places, ensuring that it strengthens bones without compromising cardiovascular health.

In addition to their roles in calcium management, Vitamin K2 and Vitamin D may also work together to support immune function. Vitamin D is known for its immune-modulating effects, helping to reduce inflammation and support the body's defense against infections. While less studied, there is some evidence to suggest that Vitamin K2 may also have anti-inflammatory properties, further enhancing the immune-supportive effects of Vitamin D. This combined action can be particularly beneficial in preventing chronic diseases that are linked to inflammation, such as cardiovascular disease and autoimmune conditions.

For individuals looking to optimize their bone and cardiovascular health, ensuring adequate intake of both Vitamin K2 and Vitamin D is essential. These vitamins are often available together in combined supplements, making it easier to achieve the right balance. However, it is also possible to obtain them through diet. Vitamin D can be synthesized by the skin in response to sunlight exposure or obtained from foods like fatty fish, fortified dairy products, and egg yolks. Vitamin K2, as discussed in previous chapters, is found in fermented foods, organ meats, and dairy products from grass-fed animals.

For those who may not get enough sunlight exposure or have difficulty consuming sufficient amounts of these nutrients through diet alone, supplementation can be a practical and effective option. It's important to choose high-quality supplements that provide both Vitamin D and Vitamin K2 in appropriate dosages, ensuring that these nutrients work together to support overall health.

In summary, the synergy between Vitamin K2 and Vitamin D highlights the importance of a balanced approach to nutrient intake. By working together, these vitamins enhance calcium absorption and utilization, protect against bone and cardiovascular diseases, and support immune function. Whether through diet, supplementation, or a combination of both, maintaining adequate levels of Vitamin K2 and Vitamin D is crucial for achieving optimal health outcomes.

Vitamin K2 and omega-3 fatty acids are two powerful nutrients that, when combined, offer significant health benefits, particularly for the heart and bones. While Vitamin K2 is primarily known for its role in calcium regulation and bone health, omega-3 fatty acids are celebrated for their anti-inflammatory properties and their ability to support cardiovascular function. Together, these nutrients create a synergistic effect that enhances overall health and helps protect against a range of chronic conditions.

Omega-3 fatty acids, which include eicosapentaenoic acid (EPA) and docosahexaenoic acid (DHA), are essential fats found in fatty fish like salmon, mackerel, and sardines, as well as in some plant-based sources such as flaxseeds and walnuts. These fatty acids play a crucial role in reducing inflammation throughout the body, which is a key factor in the development of many chronic diseases, including heart disease, arthritis, and metabolic disorders.

One of the most important benefits of omega-3s is their ability to support cardiovascular health. They help lower triglyceride levels, reduce blood pressure, and prevent the formation of blood clots, all of which are critical in reducing the risk of heart attacks and strokes. Additionally, omega-3s help maintain the health of blood vessels by enhancing their flexibility and reducing arterial stiffness, which is particularly important in preventing atherosclerosis.

When combined with Vitamin K2, the cardiovascular benefits of omega-3s are further amplified. Vitamin K2 prevents the calcification of arteries by activating matrix Gla-protein (MGP), ensuring that calcium is directed to the bones rather than the arteries. This action helps maintain arterial flexibility and reduces the risk of calcified plaques that can lead to cardiovascular events. Omega-3s, with their anti-inflammatory effects, complement this by preventing the inflammation that can damage the arterial walls and contribute to plaque formation. Together, these nutrients offer a comprehensive approach to cardiovascular protection, addressing both the inflammatory and calcification aspects of heart disease.

In addition to their cardiovascular benefits, the combination of Vitamin K2 and omega-3 fatty acids also supports bone health. While Vitamin K2 is essential for directing calcium into the bones and enhancing bone density, omega-3s play a supportive role by reducing inflammation in the joints and bones. Chronic inflammation can lead to conditions such as osteoporosis and arthritis, which weaken the bones and impair mobility. By reducing inflammation, omega-3s help create an environment that is conducive to strong, healthy bones, allowing Vitamin K2 to perform its role in calcium regulation more effectively.

Furthermore, omega-3s have been shown to support bone density by influencing the balance of bone-building and bone-resorbing cells. Omega-3s can promote the activity of osteoblasts, the cells responsible for bone formation, while inhibiting osteoclasts, the cells involved in bone resorption. This action helps maintain bone strength and density, particularly in aging populations who are at higher risk for osteoporosis.

For individuals looking to optimize their heart and bone health, incorporating both Vitamin K2 and omega-3 fatty acids into their diet or supplementation routine can be highly beneficial. Foods rich in omega-3s, such as fatty fish, should be a regular part of the diet, while Vitamin K2 can be obtained from sources like fermented foods, organ meats, and grass-fed dairy products. For those who may not consume enough of these nutrients through diet alone, high-quality supplements that provide both omega-3s and Vitamin K2 are available and can help fill any nutritional gaps.

It is also important to note that the benefits of combining Vitamin K2 with omega-3 fatty acids are not limited to heart and bone health. Both nutrients have been shown to support cognitive function, reduce the risk of chronic inflammatory diseases, and improve overall well-being. The anti-inflammatory properties of omega-3s, coupled with the calcium-regulating effects of Vitamin K2, make this combination a powerful tool for maintaining long-term health.

By focusing on a diet rich in these nutrients or choosing the right supplements, individuals can enhance their cardiovascular and bone health, reduce the risk of chronic diseases, and improve their quality of life. This synergy between Vitamin K2 and omega-3 fatty acids underscores the importance of a holistic approach to nutrition, where different nutrients work together to support overall health and prevent disease.

Balancing the intake of calcium, magnesium, and Vitamin K2 is crucial for maintaining optimal health, particularly for the health of bones and the cardiovascular system. These three nutrients work together in the body to ensure that calcium is properly absorbed, directed to the right places, and prevented from causing harm in soft tissues. Understanding how to balance these nutrients can help you make informed decisions about your diet and supplementation, ultimately supporting stronger bones and a healthier heart.

Calcium is the most abundant mineral in the body and is essential for building and maintaining strong bones and teeth. It also plays a vital role in muscle function, nerve transmission, and blood clotting. However, the benefits of calcium are largely dependent on its proper utilization within the body, which is where magnesium and Vitamin K2 come into play.

Magnesium is a critical mineral that works in concert with calcium to maintain bone health. It is involved in over 300 enzymatic reactions in the body, many of which are related to the metabolism of calcium. One of magnesium's key roles is to help convert Vitamin D into its active form, which is necessary for the absorption of calcium in the intestines. Without sufficient magnesium, calcium absorption is impaired, which can lead to lower bone density and an increased risk of fractures.

In addition to supporting calcium absorption, magnesium also plays a role in regulating calcium levels in the blood. It helps to keep calcium dissolved in the blood, preventing it from precipitating out and forming deposits in soft tissues like the arteries and kidneys. This regulation is crucial for preventing conditions such as arterial calcification and kidney stones, both of which are associated with excess calcium in the wrong places.

Vitamin K2 further enhances the balance between calcium and magnesium by ensuring that calcium is properly directed to the bones and teeth, rather than accumulating in soft tissues. Vitamin K2 activates proteins such as osteocalcin, which binds calcium to the bone matrix, and matrix Gla-protein (MGP), which inhibits calcium deposition in the arteries. This precise management of calcium is essential for maintaining bone density and preventing the calcification of arteries, a process that can lead to atherosclerosis and other cardiovascular diseases.

Achieving the right balance between calcium, magnesium, and Vitamin K2 is therefore essential for both bone and cardiovascular health. Here are some practical tips for balancing these nutrients:

- **Prioritize Dietary Sources:** Aim to get the majority of your calcium, magnesium, and Vitamin K2 from whole foods. Dairy products like milk, yogurt, and cheese are excellent sources of calcium, while leafy green vegetables, nuts, seeds, and whole grains are rich in magnesium. For Vitamin K2, focus on fermented foods, organ meats, and grass-fed dairy products.

- **Consider the Calcium-Magnesium Ratio:** It's important to maintain a healthy ratio between calcium and magnesium intake. While the ideal ratio can vary depending on individual needs, a general guideline is to aim for a 2:1 ratio of calcium to magnesium. For example, if you're consuming 1,000 mg of calcium per day, aim to get about 500 mg of magnesium.

- **Use Supplements Wisely:** If you're unable to meet your nutrient needs through diet alone, supplements can be helpful. When choosing calcium supplements, look for options that include magnesium and Vitamin K2 to ensure balanced nutrient intake. It's also important to choose high-quality supplements that are easily absorbed by the body.

- **Avoid Over-Supplementation:** While calcium, magnesium, and Vitamin K2 are essential nutrients, it's important not to over-supplement, especially with calcium. Excessive calcium intake without adequate magnesium and Vitamin K2 can lead to health issues such as kidney stones and arterial calcification. Always consult with a healthcare provider to determine the appropriate dosage for your needs.

- **Monitor Your Bone and Heart Health:** Regular check-ups that include bone density scans and cardiovascular assessments can help you track the impact of your nutrient intake on your health. This is especially important for individuals at higher risk of osteoporosis or cardiovascular disease.

By carefully balancing calcium, magnesium, and Vitamin K2, you can support strong bones, prevent the calcification of soft tissues, and reduce the risk of chronic diseases. This approach not only ensures that these nutrients work together effectively but also helps you achieve better overall health and well-being.

While supplementation can be an effective way to ensure adequate intake of essential nutrients like Vitamin K2, calcium, and magnesium, there are potential risks associated with over-supplementation. It's important to understand these risks and recognize the signs that may indicate you are consuming too much of a particular nutrient. Balancing supplementation with dietary intake and monitoring your body's response can help you avoid the pitfalls of over-supplementation and maintain optimal health.

One of the most significant risks of over-supplementation involves calcium. Calcium is crucial for bone health and various physiological functions, but too much calcium, particularly from supplements, can lead to several health issues. Excess calcium can accumulate in the blood, a condition known as hypercalcemia. Symptoms of hypercalcemia include nausea, vomiting, constipation, fatigue, and confusion. In severe cases, it can lead to kidney stones, impaired kidney function, and cardiovascular problems due to the calcification of arteries and other soft tissues.

Over-supplementing with calcium can also disrupt the balance between calcium and other minerals, such as magnesium. Magnesium is necessary for the proper metabolism of calcium, and an imbalance can lead to problems like muscle cramps, anxiety, and even more serious cardiovascular issues. If calcium levels are too high, they can outcompete magnesium for absorption, leading to magnesium deficiency, which exacerbates these symptoms.

Magnesium, while generally considered safe and less likely to cause harm in excess compared to calcium, can still pose risks if taken in very high doses, especially through supplements. Over-supplementation with magnesium can lead to gastrointestinal issues, including diarrhea, nausea, and abdominal cramping. In extremely high doses, magnesium can cause more serious side effects such as low blood pressure, irregular heartbeat, and in rare cases, cardiac arrest. These risks are generally associated with magnesium supplements rather than dietary sources, as the body can more easily regulate magnesium from food.

Vitamin K2, although less commonly associated with toxicity, can also present risks if taken in excessively high doses, particularly in individuals with certain health conditions or those taking specific medications. For example, while Vitamin K2 is generally safe and well-tolerated, individuals on anticoagulant medications (blood thinners) should be cautious, as high doses of Vitamin K2 can interfere with the medication's effectiveness. This can increase the risk of blood clots, which could lead to serious health issues such as strokes or heart attacks.

Another potential concern with over-supplementing Vitamin K2 is its interaction with other fat-soluble vitamins, particularly Vitamin A and Vitamin E. Excessive intake of one fat-soluble vitamin can interfere with the absorption and function of others, leading to imbalances and deficiencies. While this is more of a concern with synthetic forms of these vitamins, it underscores the importance of taking a balanced approach to supplementation.

Recognizing the signs of over-supplementation is key to preventing these risks. Some general signs that you may be taking too much of a particular nutrient include:

- **Gastrointestinal discomfort:** Persistent nausea, diarrhea, or constipation may indicate an imbalance or excess intake of certain supplements.
- **Fatigue and lethargy:** Feeling unusually tired or weak can be a

sign of hypercalcemia or other nutrient imbalances.
- **Muscle cramps or spasms:** These can occur if there is an imbalance between calcium and magnesium levels in the body.
- **Headaches:** Chronic headaches can sometimes be linked to over-supplementation, particularly with fat-soluble vitamins like Vitamin K2.
- **Changes in urine output or kidney function:** An increase in urinary frequency or the presence of kidney stones may indicate that your body is struggling to process excess calcium or other minerals.

To avoid the risks of over-supplementation, it is important to:

- **Consult with a healthcare provider:** Before starting any

new supplement regimen, discuss your specific needs and health conditions with a healthcare professional who can provide personalized advice on dosages and combinations.
- **Prioritize a balanced diet:** Aim to get as many nutrients as possible from whole foods, which are less likely to lead to nutrient imbalances compared to supplements.
- **Use supplements as a complement, not a substitute:** Supplements should fill in gaps in your diet, not replace healthy eating habits.
- **Follow recommended dosages:** Stick to the recommended dosages on supplement labels unless otherwise advised by a healthcare provider. Avoid the

temptation to exceed these dosages in an attempt to gain more benefits.

By being mindful of the potential risks and signs of over-supplementation, you can safely incorporate Vitamin K2, calcium, magnesium, and other nutrients into your health routine without compromising your well-being.

Incorporating Vitamin K2 into your daily health regimen, along with other essential nutrients like calcium, magnesium, and omega-3 fatty acids, requires a thoughtful approach to ensure that you achieve the best possible health outcomes. Effective supplementation strategies involve more than just taking pills; they include timing, dosage, and choosing the right combination of supplements that work together synergistically. Here are some practical tips on how to integrate Vitamin K2 with other nutrients into your daily routine.

1. Choose High-Quality Supplements

The first step in any supplementation strategy is to choose high-quality supplements from reputable brands. Look for supplements that have been third-party tested for purity and potency, ensuring that you're getting what the label claims. When selecting a Vitamin K2 supplement, consider whether it contains MK-4, MK-7, or a combination of both. MK-7 is often preferred for its longer half-life in the body, meaning it stays active longer and requires less frequent dosing. However, MK-4 is also effective, especially in supporting bone health, and may be included in comprehensive bone health supplements.

For calcium and magnesium, opt for forms that are easily absorbed by the body. Calcium citrate and magnesium glycinate are often recommended for their high bioavailability and gentle effect on the digestive system. If you're taking an omega-3 supplement, look for those that contain high levels of EPA and DHA, which are the most beneficial forms of omega-3s for heart and brain health.

2. Time Your Supplements Wisely

The timing of supplementation can impact the effectiveness of the nutrients you're taking. Vitamin K2 is fat-soluble, meaning it is best absorbed when taken with a meal that contains fat. Taking Vitamin K2 with breakfast or dinner, especially if those meals include healthy fats like olive oil, avocado, or fatty fish, can enhance its absorption.

Calcium supplements are often taken with meals as well, particularly if they are in the form of calcium carbonate, which requires stomach acid for optimal absorption. However, if you're taking calcium citrate, it can be taken with or without food. Magnesium, on the other hand, is often taken in the evening because it can have a relaxing effect on the body, helping to promote restful sleep.

If you're combining Vitamin D with Vitamin K2, consider taking them at the same time, as they work together to regulate calcium metabolism. Many supplements are now available that combine Vitamin D3 with Vitamin K2 in a single capsule, making it easier to ensure you're getting the right balance of these nutrients.

3. Start with the Right Dosages

When starting a new supplementation routine, it's important to begin with the right dosages. For Vitamin K2, the recommended daily intake can vary, but a typical dose ranges from 100 to 200 micrograms per day, depending on individual needs and health goals. Higher doses may be used in specific health conditions, but these should be guided by a healthcare provider.

For calcium, the recommended daily intake for most adults is around 1,000 to 1,200 mg, though this includes both dietary sources and supplements. If your diet is already rich in calcium, you may only need a lower-dose supplement to fill in the gaps. Magnesium intake typically ranges from 300 to 400 mg per day, depending on age and gender, but again, this includes dietary sources. Omega-3 dosages vary, but 1,000 mg of combined EPA and DHA per day is a common recommendation for general health.

4. Consider Combination Supplements

For convenience and to ensure proper nutrient balance, consider using combination supplements that provide Vitamin K2 along with other complementary nutrients. Many bone health supplements include calcium, magnesium, Vitamin D, and Vitamin K2 in a balanced formula designed to support bone density and prevent osteoporosis. Similarly, cardiovascular health supplements might combine omega-3s with Vitamin K2 and other heart-healthy nutrients like CoQ10.

These combination supplements can simplify your routine by reducing the number of separate pills you need to take while ensuring that the nutrients are provided in the correct ratios for optimal absorption and effectiveness.

5. Monitor Your Health

As you incorporate these supplements into your routine, it's important to monitor how your body responds. Keep track of any changes in your health, such as improvements in bone density, cardiovascular health, or overall well-being. Regular check-ups with your healthcare provider, including blood tests to monitor nutrient levels, can help you adjust your supplementation strategy as needed.

If you experience any adverse effects, such as digestive issues, fatigue, or unusual symptoms, consult with your healthcare provider to determine if you need to adjust the dosages or switch to different forms of the supplements.

6. Balance with a Healthy Diet

Remember that supplements are intended to complement, not replace, a healthy diet. Continue to focus on a balanced diet rich in whole foods, including plenty of vegetables, fruits, lean proteins, healthy fats, and whole grains. Foods like leafy greens, fermented products, fatty fish, nuts, and seeds can provide many of the nutrients you need, reducing your reliance on supplements.

Incorporating Vitamin K2-rich foods, such as natto, hard cheeses, and organ meats, along with calcium-rich dairy products and magnesium-rich leafy greens, will enhance your overall nutrient intake and support the effectiveness of your supplementation strategy.

By following these practical supplementation strategies, you can effectively integrate Vitamin K2 with other essential nutrients into your daily health routine. This balanced approach will help you achieve better health outcomes, supporting strong bones, a healthy heart, and overall well-being.

Creating a balanced supplement plan that includes Vitamin K2 alongside other essential nutrients like calcium, magnesium, omega-3 fatty acids, and Vitamin D can significantly enhance your health and well-being. A well-rounded approach ensures that you are not only meeting your nutritional needs but also optimizing the synergistic effects these nutrients have when they work together. This final page will guide you through the steps to build a personalized supplement plan that fits your individual health goals and lifestyle.

Assess Your Nutritional Needs

The first step in building a balanced supplement plan is to assess your current nutritional status and identify any gaps that may need to be filled through supplementation. This can be done through a combination of dietary analysis, blood tests, and a review of your health history. Understanding your baseline levels of key nutrients like Vitamin D, calcium, magnesium, and Vitamin K2 will help you determine where supplementation is most needed.

For example, if blood tests reveal that you are low in Vitamin D, it may be beneficial to start supplementing with Vitamin D3 in conjunction with Vitamin K2 to support calcium absorption and utilization. Similarly, if you have a history of osteoporosis or cardiovascular disease, focusing on calcium, magnesium, and Vitamin K2 supplementation could be critical for maintaining bone density and heart health.

Set Specific Health Goals

Your supplement plan should be tailored to your specific health goals. Whether you are looking to improve bone strength, support cardiovascular health, enhance cognitive function, or manage a chronic condition, your goals will determine which supplements are most important for you.

For instance, if your primary goal is to prevent osteoporosis, you'll want to focus on a combination of calcium, Vitamin D, and Vitamin K2, possibly along with magnesium to support bone metabolism. If heart health is your main concern, combining Vitamin K2 with omega-3 fatty acids and magnesium can help reduce the risk of arterial calcification and support healthy blood pressure levels.

Choose the Right Supplements

Once you have identified your nutritional needs and health goals, the next step is to choose high-quality supplements that meet those needs. Look for supplements that provide the nutrients you need in bioavailable forms that are easily absorbed by the body. For Vitamin K2, consider whether you prefer the MK-4 or MK-7 form, or a combination of both, depending on your health goals and any specific recommendations from your healthcare provider.

Consider combination supplements that include several of the nutrients you need in one formula. This can simplify your supplement routine and ensure that you are taking the correct ratios of nutrients. For example, a bone health supplement might include calcium, magnesium, Vitamin D, and Vitamin K2 in one capsule, providing a convenient way to meet your daily needs.

Establish a Routine

Consistency is key when it comes to supplementation. Establishing a daily routine that incorporates your supplements at the same time each day can help ensure that you don't miss doses and that your body maintains steady levels of these essential nutrients.

Consider the timing of your supplements to maximize their effectiveness. For instance, taking fat-soluble vitamins like Vitamin K2 and Vitamin D with a meal that contains healthy fats can enhance their absorption. Magnesium, which can have a calming effect, is often best taken in the evening to support relaxation and sleep.

Monitor and Adjust as Needed

As you begin your supplement plan, it's important to monitor how your body responds. Pay attention to any changes in your health, whether positive or negative, and adjust your plan as needed. Regular check-ins with your healthcare provider, including follow-up blood tests, can help you fine-tune your supplement regimen over time.

If you notice any adverse effects, such as digestive discomfort, headaches, or unusual fatigue, consult with your healthcare provider to determine whether you need to adjust your dosages or switch to different forms of supplements. It's also important to reassess your supplement plan periodically, especially if your health needs or goals change.

Complement with a Balanced Diet

Remember that supplements are intended to complement a healthy diet, not replace it. Continue to focus on a nutrient-rich diet that includes a variety of whole foods. Incorporating foods high in Vitamin K2, such as fermented products and grass-fed animal products, alongside those rich in calcium, magnesium, and omega-3s, will enhance the effectiveness of your supplement plan.

Eating a balanced diet not only helps you meet your nutritional needs but also provides additional health benefits, such as fiber, antioxidants, and phytonutrients that support overall health.

Stay Informed and Educated

Finally, staying informed about the latest research on nutrition and supplementation can help you make the best decisions for your health. As new studies emerge, you may discover additional benefits of certain nutrients or learn about new recommendations for optimal dosages. Continuing to educate yourself about your health and wellness will empower you to make informed choices that support your long-term well-being.

Building a balanced supplement plan that includes Vitamin K2 and other essential nutrients is a proactive step toward achieving and maintaining optimal health. By carefully assessing your needs, setting clear goals, choosing the right supplements, and establishing a consistent routine, you can enhance your overall health, prevent deficiencies, and support your body's natural processes for years to come.

Chapter 6: Developing a Vitamin K2 Health Plan

Understanding your individual Vitamin K2 needs is the first step in developing a personalized health plan. While Vitamin K2 is essential for everyone, the amount you need can vary based on factors such as age, diet, health conditions, and lifestyle. Assessing your Vitamin K2 needs involves taking a close look at your current health status, dietary habits, and any specific health concerns that may influence your requirements for this vital nutrient.

One of the most important factors to consider when assessing your Vitamin K2 needs is your **dietary intake**. Traditional diets rich in fermented foods, organ meats, and grass-fed animal products typically provide adequate amounts of Vitamin K2. However, modern diets, particularly those low in these foods, may result in insufficient K2 intake. If your diet lacks these sources, you may be at risk of deficiency, making it necessary to consider supplementation.

Next, consider your **bone health**. If you have a history of osteoporosis, low bone density, or frequent fractures, your Vitamin K2 needs may be higher. This is because Vitamin K2 plays a crucial role in directing calcium to the bones, where it can strengthen and maintain bone density. Women, especially postmenopausal women, are often at higher risk for bone density issues and may benefit from increased Vitamin K2 intake.

Cardiovascular health is another critical factor. Vitamin K2 helps prevent the calcification of arteries, which can lead to atherosclerosis and other heart-related issues. If you have a history of heart disease, high blood pressure, or other cardiovascular concerns, ensuring adequate Vitamin K2 intake can be an essential part of your health plan. Regular cardiovascular assessments, such as blood pressure monitoring and cholesterol checks, can help you determine whether your Vitamin K2 intake needs adjustment.

Your **age** also plays a role in determining your Vitamin K2 needs. As we age, the body's ability to absorb and utilize certain nutrients can decline, making it more challenging to maintain optimal levels through diet alone. Older adults may require higher Vitamin K2 intake to support bone and cardiovascular health. Additionally, the natural decline in bone density and the increased risk of arterial calcification with age further emphasize the importance of adequate Vitamin K2.

For individuals with **specific health conditions** such as diabetes, chronic kidney disease, or metabolic syndrome, Vitamin K2 can play a supportive role in managing these conditions. For example, Vitamin K2's ability to improve insulin sensitivity and regulate glucose metabolism makes it beneficial for those with diabetes. If you have any chronic health conditions, consider how Vitamin K2 might fit into your broader treatment plan.

Finally, assess your **lifestyle** and how it may impact your Vitamin K2 needs. Factors such as high levels of physical activity, stress, and exposure to environmental toxins can increase your body's demand for essential nutrients, including Vitamin K2. Athletes, in particular, may benefit from higher Vitamin K2 intake to support bone strength and recovery from intense physical activity.

To accurately assess your Vitamin K2 needs, consider keeping a **dietary log** for a week to track your intake of K2-rich foods. This can provide valuable insights into whether you are getting enough of this nutrient from your diet or if supplementation is necessary. You can also discuss your dietary habits and health concerns with a healthcare provider, who can recommend appropriate blood tests to check your Vitamin K2 status and provide personalized advice on supplementation.

By carefully assessing your Vitamin K2 needs, you can create a foundation for a health plan that supports your overall well-being and addresses your specific health concerns. This personalized approach ensures that you are taking the right steps to maintain optimal levels of Vitamin K2 and reap the full benefits of this important nutrient.

Setting clear and achievable health goals is essential when incorporating Vitamin K2 into your health plan. These goals will guide your actions and help you track progress as you work towards improving your overall well-being. Whether your focus is on bone health, cardiovascular support, or general wellness, having specific goals can make your Vitamin K2 regimen more effective and tailored to your needs.

To begin, think about your **primary health concerns**. For many people, maintaining strong bones is a top priority, particularly as they age. If bone health is your focus, your goals might include improving bone density, reducing the risk of fractures, or supporting recovery from bone-related injuries. In this case, you might aim to increase your intake of Vitamin K2-rich foods or consider a supplement that supports bone mineralization and density.

If your concern is **heart health**, you might set goals around maintaining healthy arteries and preventing calcification. This could involve regular cardiovascular assessments to monitor the condition of your arteries, along with integrating Vitamin K2 into your daily routine to support arterial health. Your goals could also include lifestyle adjustments, such as incorporating more heart-healthy activities like regular exercise and a balanced diet that complements your Vitamin K2 intake.

For those interested in **overall wellness**, Vitamin K2 can be part of a broader goal to enhance vitality and prevent age-related conditions. In this context, your goals might focus on maintaining energy levels, improving metabolic health, or supporting skin and dental health. You might set specific targets, such as including more fermented foods in your diet, which are naturally high in Vitamin K2, or establishing a consistent supplementation routine that fits seamlessly into your lifestyle.

When setting your goals, it's important to make them **specific, measurable, and realistic**. For example, instead of a general goal like "improve bone health," you might set a more specific goal like "increase bone density by 5% over the next year." This gives you a clear target to work towards and allows you to measure your progress with tools like bone density scans or other health assessments.

Additionally, consider the **time frame** for your goals. Some health improvements, such as increased bone density or reduced arterial calcification, may take several months or even years to achieve. Setting both short-term and long-term goals can help you stay motivated and see the progress you're making over time. For instance, a short-term goal might be to start incorporating a daily Vitamin K2 supplement within the next month, while a long-term goal could be to achieve a certain health milestone by the end of the year.

Consistency is key to reaching your goals. Once you've established your objectives, commit to a regular routine that includes the necessary dietary and lifestyle changes to support your Vitamin K2 intake. This might involve setting reminders to take your supplements, planning meals that include K2-rich foods, or scheduling regular check-ups to monitor your health progress.

Finally, don't forget to **celebrate your successes**. Achieving your health goals, no matter how small, is a significant step towards better health. Acknowledging your progress can help reinforce positive habits and keep you motivated as you continue to work towards your larger health objectives.

By setting clear and actionable goals, you create a roadmap for incorporating Vitamin K2 into your health plan, ensuring that you can effectively track your progress and achieve the health outcomes that matter most to you.

Monitoring your progress is an essential part of any health plan, especially when integrating Vitamin K2 into your routine. Tracking how your body responds to

Vitamin K2 will help you determine whether your current intake is effective or if adjustments are needed to better meet your health goals. By regularly assessing your progress, you can make informed decisions that ensure you're getting the most out of your supplementation or dietary changes.

To effectively track your progress, start by identifying key **health indicators** that align with your goals. If your focus is on bone health, for example, regular bone density scans can provide valuable insights into how your bones are responding to increased Vitamin K2 intake. These scans can show changes in bone mineral density over time, helping you assess whether your Vitamin K2 levels are adequate or if adjustments are needed to further improve bone strength.

For those concentrating on cardiovascular health, tracking progress might involve **monitoring arterial health**. This can be done through regular blood pressure checks, cholesterol levels, and other cardiovascular assessments recommended by your healthcare provider. If you're aiming to prevent or reduce arterial calcification, periodic scans that assess the condition of your arteries can help you see the impact of Vitamin K2 on your cardiovascular system.

Symptom tracking is another effective way to monitor how Vitamin K2 is affecting your health. Keep a journal of any symptoms related to your health goals, such as joint pain, muscle cramps, or skin condition changes. Over time, you may notice improvements that correspond with your Vitamin K2 intake, which can indicate that your current regimen is working well. Conversely, if symptoms persist or worsen, it may be a sign that adjustments are necessary.

In addition to physical assessments, consider tracking your **energy levels, mood, and overall well-being**. These more subjective measures can provide important clues about how your body is responding to Vitamin K2. For example, if you find that your energy levels are consistently higher or that you're experiencing fewer mood swings, it could suggest that your Vitamin K2 intake is positively influencing your overall health.

Adjusting your Vitamin K2 intake is sometimes necessary based on the progress you observe. If your bone density scans show only minimal improvement, or if cardiovascular assessments indicate ongoing arterial calcification, you might need to increase your intake of Vitamin K2. This could involve taking a higher dose of supplements, incorporating more K2-rich foods into your diet, or even considering different forms of Vitamin K2 (such as MK-4 or MK-7) that might be more effective for your specific health needs.

On the other hand, if you notice signs of over-supplementation, such as gastrointestinal discomfort or unusual fatigue, it may be necessary to reduce your intake. It's important to listen to your body and consult with a healthcare provider to adjust your dosage accordingly.

Regular consultations with your healthcare provider are crucial when tracking progress and adjusting your intake. Your provider can offer professional guidance based on your health assessments, blood tests, and any symptoms you're experiencing. They can also help you navigate any challenges that arise and ensure that your Vitamin K2 plan remains aligned with your overall health strategy.

To stay organized, consider using **tracking tools** such as apps or spreadsheets to record your progress. These tools can help you keep all your health data in one place, making it easier to spot trends and make informed decisions. Whether it's tracking your daily supplement intake, noting changes in symptoms, or recording the results of health assessments, having a centralized system can streamline the process and keep you on track.

By regularly tracking your progress and being open to adjusting your Vitamin K2 intake as needed, you can ensure that your health plan remains effective and responsive to your body's needs. This proactive approach will help you achieve your health goals more efficiently and maintain optimal well-being over the long term.

Incorporating Vitamin K2 into your daily routine doesn't have to be complicated. With a few practical strategies, you can easily make Vitamin K2 a consistent part of your lifestyle, whether through diet, supplementation, or a combination of both. The key is to create habits that fit seamlessly into your existing routines, ensuring that you reap the full benefits of this essential nutrient.

One of the simplest ways to increase your Vitamin K2 intake is by **adding K2-rich foods to your meals**. Fermented foods like natto, sauerkraut, and certain cheeses are excellent sources of Vitamin K2, particularly in its MK-7 form. Including these foods in your diet can be as easy as adding a spoonful of sauerkraut to your lunch or enjoying a slice of cheese with your breakfast. For those who enjoy trying new things, natto—a traditional Japanese fermented soybean dish—can be a powerful addition to your diet, though it may take some time to get used to its strong flavor and texture.

Animal products from grass-fed sources, such as liver, egg yolks, and butter, are also rich in Vitamin K2, especially the MK-4 form. Incorporating these into your meals can be straightforward—consider cooking with grass-fed butter, adding a boiled egg to your salad, or preparing liver once a week as part of your dinner rotation. These small adjustments can significantly boost your Vitamin K2 intake without requiring major changes to your diet.

If your diet alone doesn't provide enough Vitamin K2, **supplementation can be an effective way to meet your needs**. Choose a supplement that fits easily into your routine. Many Vitamin K2 supplements are available in combination with other nutrients like Vitamin D, which is particularly convenient if you're also looking to support bone or cardiovascular health. Taking your supplement at the same time each day—such as with your breakfast or dinner—can help establish a habit that's easy to maintain.

To make Vitamin K2 supplementation even more seamless, consider setting up **automated reminders**. Whether it's a daily alarm on your phone or a pill organizer that you check each morning, these tools can ensure that you don't forget to take your supplement, especially on busy days. If you travel frequently, keeping a small supply of your supplements in a travel-friendly container can help you stay on track while on the go.

Incorporating Vitamin K2 into your lifestyle also involves **making mindful choices at the grocery store**. When shopping, look for foods that are naturally high in Vitamin K2, and consider selecting organic or grass-fed options when possible, as these tend to have higher K2 content. Reading labels and becoming familiar with brands that offer K2-rich products can make your shopping trips more efficient and help you consistently choose the best options for your health.

Meal planning can be another effective strategy for integrating Vitamin K2 into your daily life. By planning your meals ahead of time, you can ensure that you're including a variety of K2-rich foods throughout the week. This approach not only supports consistent K2 intake but also helps you maintain a balanced diet overall. For example, you might plan to have a spinach salad with boiled eggs on Monday, a serving of liver with vegetables on Wednesday, and a cheese plate as a weekend snack. By spreading these foods out over the week, you can enjoy a diverse and nutrient-rich diet without feeling overwhelmed.

For those who are more socially inclined, consider **sharing your Vitamin K2 journey with friends or family**. Cooking meals together that include K2-rich ingredients or discussing the benefits of Vitamin K2 can make the process more enjoyable and encourage others to join you in prioritizing their health. This shared experience can help reinforce your own habits and create a supportive environment for maintaining your health goals.

Finally, remember that integrating Vitamin K2 into your life is not just about meeting your nutritional needs—it's also about building a sustainable and enjoyable routine that enhances your overall well-being. By making small, consistent changes and finding ways to incorporate K2-rich foods and supplements into your existing habits, you can ensure that Vitamin K2 becomes a natural and beneficial part of your daily life.

Maintaining consistent Vitamin K2 intake can present a few challenges, especially for those who are new to supplementation or have dietary restrictions. However, with some practical solutions and a bit of planning, these challenges can be easily managed, ensuring that you can maintain optimal levels of Vitamin K2 and support your health goals effectively.

One of the most common challenges is **remembering to take supplements consistently**. Life gets busy, and it's easy to forget a dose, especially when starting a new supplement regimen. To overcome this, consider incorporating your supplements into a routine that's already well-established. For example, if you have a morning routine that includes brushing your teeth and having breakfast, place your Vitamin K2 supplement near your toothbrush or in the kitchen where you prepare your meal. This visual reminder can help reinforce the habit until it becomes second nature.

Another helpful strategy is to use **technology** to your advantage. Set daily reminders on your smartphone or use a health app that tracks your supplement intake. These tools can send you notifications at a specific time each day, ensuring that you don't miss a dose. For those who prefer a more hands-on approach, a pill organizer with compartments for each day of the week can also be a useful tool, making it easy to see if you've taken your supplement for the day.

For individuals with **dietary restrictions**, such as vegetarians or those with food allergies, finding Vitamin K2-rich foods can be more challenging. Natto, a fermented soybean product, is one of the richest sources of Vitamin K2 and is suitable for vegetarians, but its strong taste may not appeal to everyone. In such cases, it may be beneficial to explore other fermented foods like sauerkraut, miso, or certain cheeses that are also good sources of K2. If these foods are not part of your diet, or if you have allergies that limit your options, a high-quality Vitamin K2 supplement can help fill the gap.

Another challenge is **ensuring the right balance with other nutrients**, such as calcium, magnesium, and Vitamin D. It's important to remember that these nutrients work synergistically, and imbalances can affect how well they function in the body. To overcome this, consider using combination supplements that include Vitamin K2 along with these other key nutrients. This not only simplifies your supplementation routine but also ensures that you're getting the right ratios of each nutrient for optimal health benefits.

For those who travel frequently or have an unpredictable schedule, **staying consistent with supplementation** can be particularly challenging. In this case, it's helpful to keep a small, portable supply of your supplements in your bag or car. Travel-sized pill containers or pre-packaged supplement packets can make it easier to maintain your routine while on the go. Additionally, setting a specific time of day for taking your supplements, such as during breakfast or dinner, can help create consistency even when your environment changes.

Financial considerations can also be a barrier for some individuals when it comes to maintaining a consistent supplement regimen. High-quality supplements can be expensive, and not everyone has the budget to buy them regularly. To manage this, look for cost-effective options, such as buying in bulk or choosing a subscription service that offers discounts for regular purchases. Additionally, focusing on food sources of Vitamin K2 can help reduce reliance on supplements, potentially lowering costs. Shopping for seasonal or locally produced K2-rich foods can also be a more affordable way to meet your needs.

Finally, if you're experiencing **side effects** or discomfort from supplementation, it's important to address these issues promptly. Some people may experience mild digestive upset or other side effects when they first start taking a new supplement. If this happens, try taking your supplement with food or dividing the dose into smaller amounts throughout the day. If side effects persist, consult with a healthcare provider to adjust your dosage or explore alternative forms of the supplement that may be better tolerated.

By anticipating these challenges and implementing strategies to overcome them, you can maintain consistent Vitamin K2 intake and continue working towards your health goals without disruption. With the right approach, Vitamin K2 supplementation can become a seamless part of your daily routine, providing you with the benefits of this essential nutrient for years to come.

Incorporating Vitamin K2 into your long-term health strategy is a powerful way to support your overall well-being. As you've learned throughout this chapter, Vitamin K2 plays a crucial role in maintaining bone density, preventing arterial calcification, and contributing to various other aspects of health. The key to maximizing these benefits is to make Vitamin K2 a consistent and sustainable part of your daily life, ensuring that your body receives the support it needs over time.

When planning for the long term, it's important to view Vitamin K2 as part of a broader approach to health. This includes balancing your diet with a variety of nutrient-rich foods, engaging in regular physical activity, and maintaining healthy lifestyle habits. By integrating these elements, you can create a comprehensive health plan that not only supports your immediate goals but also promotes lasting vitality.

Consistency is crucial when it comes to reaping the full benefits of Vitamin K2. Whether you're obtaining it from food, supplements, or a combination of both, maintaining regular intake is essential for supporting bone health and preventing calcification in your arteries. Establishing routines, such as taking your supplements at the same time each day or planning meals that include K2-rich foods, can help you stay on track.

Monitoring your health over time is another key component of long-term planning. Regular check-ups with your healthcare provider, including bone density scans and cardiovascular assessments, will help you track the effectiveness of your Vitamin K2 regimen and make adjustments as needed. These assessments provide valuable feedback, allowing you to fine-tune your approach and ensure that you're meeting your health goals.

As part of your long-term strategy, it's also important to **stay informed** about new research and developments related to Vitamin K2 and overall health. The field of nutrition is constantly evolving, and staying updated can help you make informed decisions about your supplementation and dietary choices. Consider subscribing to reputable health newsletters, following experts in the field, or discussing the latest findings with your healthcare provider.

Adapting your plan as your needs change is another essential aspect of long-term health planning. As you age, your nutritional requirements may shift, or you may develop new health goals. Being flexible and willing to adjust your Vitamin K2 intake, along with other aspects of your health plan, will help you continue to meet your body's needs effectively. For example, if you experience changes in bone density or cardiovascular health, you may need to increase your intake of Vitamin K2 or explore different forms of supplementation.

Finally, consider **sharing your knowledge and experience** with others. Whether it's family, friends, or community groups, discussing the benefits of Vitamin K2 and how it fits into a healthy lifestyle can help raise awareness and encourage others to take proactive steps for their health. This not only reinforces your own commitment but also creates a supportive environment where healthy habits can thrive.

In conclusion, developing a long-term health plan that includes Vitamin K2 is an investment in your future well-being. By committing to consistent intake, monitoring your progress, staying informed, and being adaptable, you can harness the full potential of this vital nutrient to support your bones, heart, and overall health for years to come.

Made in United States
North Haven, CT
15 November 2024